DIABETIC AIR FRYER COOKBOOK

Discover All The Best Secrets To Prepare Healthy Air Fryer Fried Food With Low Fat, Low Sugar, And Low Carb for A Healthy Delicious Type 1 and Type 2 Diabetics Diet.

by Sarah Bravekins

Table of Contents

Introduction

Diabetic Air-Fry Cookbook is a kind of handbook, which will tell you how to make delicious food with an Air Fryer without compromising its taste. It is a cool book for health-conscious people because it provides recipes, which are 100% healthy and at the same time tasty. Diabetic Air-Fry Cookbook has been released in e-book edition rather than the traditional paper form so that it can be available to all people across the globe.

If you are a family member of someone with diabetes or you're a healthy companion, try Diabetic Air-Fry Cookbook for some tasty food, and feel free to contact me any time if you have anything to comment or suggest.

An Air Fryer is a new method of deep frying food at home. It is the latest home appliances that has been developed. With this machine, you can easily cook delicious dishes at home in the shortest time. There are several models available in the market. Before going to buy, it's better to know about its operating modes and other features. So here we discuss the things to know before buying a deep fryer.

It is very easy to use and healthier. You can prepare all your favorite dishes with less oil, which is not good for your health. With this machine, you can make different kinds of food such as baked foods, dumplings, fried snacks, etc. This appliance helps you to save your precious time.

This easy cookbook takes you through the process of making great tasting food, but without any hesitation. You'll be delighted by the flavors you create in your home. This wonderful cookbook is filled with tips, tricks, and pointers that will make your air-fryer come alive!

Diabetes is by far the fastest-growing disease in the world. Experts predict that the number of diabetics could hit 2 billion by 2050. That's a shocking thought, but what can we do to help?

The answer may be found in an air-fryer (also known as "air-tight fryers") which is a new cooking appliance that allows you to cook foods quickly and easily without oils. It's perfect for people with diabetes because it cooks foods without adding any carbohydrates or oils to them at all. Unlike other similar appliances, it requires no electricity to operate.

In this cookbook, we'll teach you everything you need to know about using an air-fryer. Cook food quickly and easily without oil! Unlike other types of appliances that use oils or fats, which burn easily during cooking and end up giving your food a greasy taste…The air-fryer doesn't! Because the food is cooked in hot air, it stays healthier than foods cooked with oil or fats. There are no oils or fats added during cooking… Just hot air! Cooking time can be drastically cut down because all you have to do is set your timer and leave it alone! You can cook many different kind of foods at once because there's no oil or fat involved, you can cook everything. Using an air-fryer is easy! Like most things, it takes practice until you get it right. Find out how to fill the air-fryer with the right amount of oil, and use the right temperature for the right time. We've listed all of our top tips and tricks in this book, so you can cook like a pro.

Are you a diabetic that loves to cook? It is very important to eat well when you have diabetes, and air-fryers are the best way to do so. This book contains solutions to all of your problems! Air-frying is a great way to prepare food without using a lot of oil. Most people think that they need to fill their air-fryer with oil every time they use it, and this can cause some problems. When you are only using a small amount of oil for a large amount of food, you will save money on your next meal! Plus, it's great for the environment! All you need is just about any food that would normally need oil. Garlic, potatoes, or even meat would be perfect for an air-fryer. You will still get the same great taste without having to use much oil at all! (You can tell we like air-fries!)

Chapter 1. What is, How to Use and How to Clean an Air- Fryer?

What Is an Air Fryer?

The Air Fryer has become the most popular and trendy kitchen appliance this year. But why are people excited about it? Why has it become a favorite of people who love fried food? Why is it promoting frying being healthy? The Air Fryer is nothing like a typical deep fryer. This cooking utensil is much more like a small, stylish and self-contained oven that uses a convection cooking method. It uses an electrical element that heats the air in the fryer and then circulates it evenly around the food for its cooking. As a result, this hot air cooks the food in the fryer quickly and brings out the well-cooked food that is evenly browned and crunchy on the outside, but the inside of the food stays moist and tasty.

How to Use an Air-Fryer?

Here's how you can start cooking with your Air Fryer and get most of it.

Adjust the Cooking Temperature

Although there are many air frying recipes and at the beginning of your Air Fryer cooking, you should stick to them to understand how Air Fryer cooking works and how proficient in air frying cooking is. Then, move on to convert your regular deep frying or oven-baked recipes into air frying one. For this, reduce the cooking temperature by 25 ⁰F to achieve the same result in terms of texture and taste of your food. For example, if your recipe is deep-fried in the oil heated to 350 ⁰F, then Air Fryer cooks the same food at 325 ⁰F. This rule applies to other converting recipes, be it baking, roasting, broiling, etc. Remember to preheat your Air Fryer to temperature 220 ⁰F or recipe suggested temperature, it usually takes 5 minutes, and then fill the frying basket for further cooking.

Toss the Ingredients with Oil

Although the Air Fryer's cooking accessories are non-stick, you should still toss your food ingredients in oil, about 1 to 2 tablespoons. You can skip this step for foods that are naturally fatty, like meatballs. For foods that are coated in flour or battered, cook them in the greased frying basket and then coat the top of the food with an oil spray. This oil is essential to make sure that air fried food turns out golden-brown, crunchy and appealing.

Filling the Frying Basket

Foods coated with flour or battered should be fry in one layer in the Air Fryer. For foods like fries or vegetables, you can load the frying basket to the top, but a full basket takes a long cooking time and may result in food that is not quite crispy. It is also recommended to shake the basket at least twice to make sure food is cook evenly.

Check the Doneness Early

Circulation of hot air in the Air Fryer helps in maintaining a consistent temperature in the Air Fryer, which cooks the food faster than being cooked in a conventional oven and deep fryer. This worth that if you are adapting your regular food into an Air Fryer one or the recipe you have already cooked in an Air Fryer, you will need to check the food about two-third of the suggested cooking time to test its doneness. For example, if the fish sticks recipe says to be cooked in 15 minutes, then start checking them at 10 minutes.

How to Clean an Air-Fryer?

Air Fryers can give you crispier foods that satisfy your cravings, and, as we conclude, here are a few tips to ensure success while using your Air Fryer. Here are certain tips for you to get the most out of your Air Fryer:

1. **Shake it frequently while cooking**: be sure to open the fryer and shake what you are cooking around as they "fry" in the basket. Smaller foods, such as French fries and chips may compress. Even if a recipe does not mention to rotate, shake, or flip, make sure to do so every 5-10 minutes for the best results.

2. **Do not overcrowd food while cooking:** make sure you give foods lots of space for the hot air to circulate effectively around what you are cooking. This will give you the crispy results you crave! Also, it is best to work in small batches.

3. **Secure foods**: on occasion, your Air Fryer will pick up foods that are light and blow them around the fryer. Secure foods you cook with toothpicks!

4. **Check your food's doneness frequently**: one of the best benefits of cooking with an Air Fryer is that you do not have to worry about how often you open it up to check for doneness. If you are an anxious chef, this can give you peace of mind to create yummy meals and snacks every single time!

5. **Take out basket before removing food**: if you go to invert the Air Fryer basket when it is still locked tightly in the drawer, you will dump all the fat that has been rendered from your food.

6. **Clean the drawer after each use:** the Air Fryer drawer is extremely easy to clean and quite hassle-free. But if you leave it unwashed, you can risk contaminating the future food you cook, and you may have a nasty smell take over your kitchen. Simply clean it after every use to prevent this.

7. **Use the air dryer to dry the appliance out**: after you wash the basket and Air Fryer drawer, you can pop them back into the fryer and turn on the appliance for 2-3 minutes. This is a great way to dry it for your next use thoroughly!

Chapter 2. What Is Diabetes?

According to the CDC, over 30 million individuals in America have diabetes; and 1 in 4 of these people don't know they have this condition. The cause of diabetes is linked with the pancreases, which cannot produce or use insulin properly. Insulin hormone is stashed into the bloodstream by the pancreatic gland to deliver it into the cells. Once the cells take in the sugar, it is converted into energy and used immediately or stored for later use.

Differences between Type 1 and 2 Diabetes

Type 1 Diabetes

It is a sugar dependent on insulin treatment and usually affects young children and young adults under 20 years, and this type is characterized by the inability of the pancreas to produce insulin.

This type requires:

- Insulin.

- Diet food.

- Sports.

It is essential for patients to understand that this type does not respond to treatment with cereals.

Type 2 Diabetes

Type 2 diabetes is the most common type and makes up 90% of people with diabetes. This type is called insulin-dependent diabetes, and it is the most prevalent type in adults over 40 years old or overweight. Sometimes it affects children over ten years old and occurs as a result of the body's inability to secrete enough insulin or an adequate amount of the hormone insulin, but it is ineffective, resulting in high blood sugar.

Only about 50% of patients with diabetes are diagnosed because there are few and insufficient symptoms or some similar symptoms to other diseases in the early stages of the disease.

If left untreated, the disease will lead to vision loss, heart attacks, strokes, and kidney failure.

This type requires:

- Diet.

- Sports.

- Pills.

Are There Any Genetic Causes for Type 2 Diabetes?

The genetic factor has a role in the specific transmission of diabetes. But clearly, diabetes type2 depends in large part on the presence of genetic predisposition more than about it in type 1 diabetes:

In the case of identical twins (from one egg), if a brother develops type 2 diabetes, then there is a possibility his brother's injury is 60-90%.

Having a family history for one person with type 2 diabetes increases the incidence rate twice, and having a family history for two people increases the incidence rate 4 times.

Causes of injury:

- Automatic immunity against insulin.

- Obesity and overweight.

- Exposure to viral infections (mumps or pancreatitis).

- What are the normal proportions of blood sugar level?

- The rate of normal sugar blood (Fasting) (80 - 100 mg/dl).

- The rate of normal sugar blood (Two hours after eating) (less than 140 mg/dl).

- What is the percentage of blood sugar that means an increased chance of diabetes (pre-diabetes)?

- The rate of sugar (fasting) is between (100 - 125 mg/dl).

- Concentrated glucose tolerance test, i.e., giving the patient (75 mg) of concentrated glucose fluid and checking blood sugar after two hours' equals between (140 - 199 mg/dl).

It means increasing the chance of developing diabetes more in the future. In this case, a schedule of your own will be set up by the primary health care physician to do a blood sugar check periodically.

There are other types of diabetes such as:

- Gestational Diabetes

- Secondary diabetes that is resulted in:

  o Chronic pancreatic disease (Chronic Inflammation)

  o Endocrine disorders such as Giant disease and Cushing's disease

  o Use of certain medications, such as cortisone.

Recommended Foods and Foods to Avoid

Food Group / Enjoy Freely	Eat In Moderation (Limited to < 1 Serving)	Avoid Or Limit
Dairy Nonfat And 1%-Fat Milk, Low-Fat And Nonfat Cheese, Low-Fat And Nonfat Yogurt, Low-Fat And Nonfat Cottage Cheese, Low-Fat And Nonfat Ricotta Cheese, Nonfat Cream Cheese, Nonfat Sour Cream	2%-Fat Milk (8 Ounces), Low-Fat Cream Cheese (1 Tablespoon), Low-Fat Sour Cream (1 Tablespoon)	Whole Milk, Full-Fat Cheese, Regular Sour Cream, Regular Cream Cheese, Full-Fat Yogurt
Fruits Citrus, Berries, Bananas, Grapes, Melons, Pineapples, Mangos, Peaches, Apricots, Apples, Pears, Plums, Kiwis	Avocado (½), Dried Fruit (¼ Cup)	None
Grains Whole Wheat And Whole-Grain Breads, Whole-Grain	White Bread (1 Slice), White Pasta (½ Cup	Sugar-Filled Breakfast Cereals,

Breakfast Cereals, Wheat Germ, Brown Rice, Bulgur, Whole Wheat Couscous, Quinoa, Oatmeal	Cooked), White Rice (½ Cup Cooked)	Donuts, Pastries, Cakes, Cookies, Pies
Fats And Oils Canola Oil, Olive Oil, Vegetable Oil	Butter (1 Teaspoon), Mayonnaise (1 Tablespoon), Salad Dressing (1 Tablespoon)	Coconut Oil, Palm Oil, Lard, Solid Margarine
Proteins Lean Poultry, Fish, Eggs, Beans, Legumes, Tofu	Nuts And Seeds(1/3 cup of Nuts), 2 Tablespoons Of Seeds, 2 Tablespoons Of Nut Butter), Red Meat (6 Ounces Or Fewer)	Bacon, Sausage, Hot Dogs, Luncheon Meats, And Smoked, Cured, Or Pickled Foods
Vegetables: Tomatoes, Carrots, Summer Squash, Broccoli, Leafy Greens, Mushrooms, Green Beans, Cabbage, Cauliflower, Asparagus, Brussels Sprouts, Onions	Winter Squash (½ Cup), Corn (½ Cup), Green Peas (2/3 cup)	None

Chapter 3. Protein Recipes

Parmesan Shrimp

Preparation Time: 10 minutes

Cooking Time: 10 minutes

Servings: 6

Ingredients:

- 2 pounds jumbo shrimp, wild-caught, peeled, deveined

- 2 tablespoons of minced garlic

- 1 teaspoon of onion powder

- 1 teaspoon of basil

- 1 teaspoon of ground black pepper

- 1/2 teaspoon of dried oregano

- 2 tablespoons of olive oil

- 2/3 cup of grated Parmesan cheese, reduced-fat

- 2 tablespoons of lemon juice

Directions:

1. Switch on the Air Fryer, insert the fryer basket, grease it with olive oil, then shut with its lid, set the fryer to 350 °F, and preheat for 5 minutes.

2. Meanwhile, place cheese in a bowl, add remaining ingredients except for shrimps and lemon juice and stir until combined.

3. Add shrimps and then toss until well coated.

4. Open the fryer, add shrimps in it, spray oil over them, close with its lid and cook for 10 minutes until nicely golden and crispy, shaking halfway through the frying.

5. When the Air Fryer beeps, open its lid, transfer chicken onto a serving plate, drizzle with lemon juice and serve.

Nutrition:

- Calories: 307 Cal

- Carbs: 12 g

- Fat: 16.4 g

- Protein: 27.6 g

- Fiber: 3 g

Tilapia

Preparation Time: 5 minutes

Cooking Time: 12 minutes

Servings: 2

Ingredients:

- 2 tilapia fillets, wild-caught, 1 ½ inch thick

- 1 teaspoon of old bay seasoning

- ¾ teaspoon of lemon pepper seasoning

- ½ teaspoon of salt

Directions:

1. Switch on the Air Fryer, insert fryer basket, grease it with olive oil, then shut with its lid, set the fryer to 400°F, and preheat for 5 minutes.

2. Meanwhile, spray tilapia fillets with oil and then season with salt, lemon, pepper, and old bay seasoning until evenly coated.

3. Open the fryer, add tilapia in it, close with its lid and cook for 7 minutes until nicely golden and cooked, turning the fillets halfway through the frying.

4. When the Air Fryer beeps, open its lid, transfer tilapia fillets onto a serving plate and serve.

Nutrition:

- Calories: 36 Cal

- Carbs: 0 g

- Fat: 0.75 g

- Protein: 7.4 g

- Fiber: 0 g

Tomato Basil Scallops

Preparation Time: 5 minutes

Cooking Time: 15 minutes

Servings: 2

Ingredients:

- 8 jumbo sea scallops, wild-caught

- 1 tablespoon of tomato paste

- 12 ounces of frozen spinach, thawed and drained

- 1 tablespoon of chopped fresh basil

- 1 teaspoon of ground black pepper

- 1 teaspoon of minced garlic

- 1 teaspoon of salt

- 3/4 cup of heavy whipping cream, reduced-fat

Directions:

1. Switch on the Air Fryer, insert fryer basket, grease it with olive oil, then shut with its lid, set the fryer to 350°F, and preheat for 5 minutes.

2. Meanwhile, take a 7 inches baking pan, grease it with oil, and place spinach in it in an even layer.

3. Spray the scallops with oil, sprinkle with ½ teaspoon each of salt and black pepper, and then place scallops over the spinach.

4. Place tomato paste in a bowl, whisk in cream, basil, garlic, and remaining salt and black pepper until smooth, and then pour over the scallops.

5. Open the fryer, place the pan in it, close with its lid, and cook for 10 minutes until thoroughly cooked and sauce is hot.

6. Serve straight away.

Nutrition:

- Calories: 359 Cal

- Carbs: 6 g

- Fat: 33 g

- Protein: 9 g

- Fiber: 1 g

Shrimp Scampi

Preparation Time: 5 minutes

Cooking Time: 12 minutes

Servings: 4

Ingredients:

- 1-pound shrimp, peeled, deveined

- 1 tablespoon of minced garlic

- 1 tablespoon of minced basil

- 1 tablespoon of lemon juice

- 1 teaspoon of dried chives

- 1 teaspoon of dried basil

- 2 teaspoons of red pepper flakes

- 4 tablespoons of butter, unsalted

- 2 tablespoons of chicken stock

Directions:

1. Switch on the Air Fryer, insert fryer pan, grease it with olive oil, then shut with its lid, set the fryer to 330°F, and preheat for 5 minutes.

2. Add butter in it along with red pepper and garlic and cook for 2 minutes or until the butter has melted.

3. Then add remaining ingredients in the pan, stir until mixed and continue cooking for 5 minutes until shrimps have cooked, stirring halfway through.

4. When done, remove the pan from the Air Fryer, stir the shrimp scampi, let it rest for 1 minute and then stir again.

5. Garnish shrimps with basil leaves and serve.

Nutrition:

- Calories: 221 Cal

- Carbs: 1 g

- Fat: 13 g

- Protein: 23 g

- Fiber: 0 g

Salmon Cakes

Preparation Time: 5 minutes

Cooking Time: 12 minutes

Servings: 2

Ingredients:

- ½ cup of almond flour

- 15 ounces of cooked pink salmon

- ¼ teaspoon of ground black pepper

- 2 teaspoons of Dijon mustard

- 2 tablespoons of chopped fresh dill

- 2 tablespoons of mayonnaise, reduced-fat

- 1 egg, pastured

- 2 wedges of lemon

Directions:

1. Switch on the Air Fryer, insert fryer basket, grease it with olive oil, then shut with its lid, set the fryer to ⊄00°F, and preheat for 5 minutes.

2. Meanwhile, place all the ingredients in a bowl, except for lemon wedges, stir until combined, and then shape into four patties, each about 4-inches.

3. Open the fryer, add salmon patties in it, spray oil over them, close with its lid and cook for 12 minutes until nicely golden and crispy, flipping the patties halfway through the frying.

4. When the Air Fryer beeps, open its lid, transfer salmon patties onto a serving plate and serve.

Nutrition:

- Calories: 517 Cal

- Carbs: 15 g

- Fat: 27 g

- Protein: 52 g

- Fiber: 5 g

Tex-Mex Salmon Stir-Fry

Preparation Time: 15 Minutes

Cooking Time: 9 to 14 Minutes

Servings: 4

Ingredients:

- 12 ounces of salmon fillets, cut into 1½-inch cubes (see Tip)

- 1 red bell pepper, chopped

- 1 red onion, chopped

- 1 jalapeño pepper, minced

- ¼ cup of low-sodium salsa

- 2 tablespoons of low-sodium tomato juice

- 2 teaspoons of peanut oil or safflower oil

- 1 teaspoon of chili powder

- Brown rice or polenta, cooked (optional)

Directions:

1. In an intermediate bowl, blend the salmon, red bell pepper, red onion, jalapeño, salsa, tomato juice, peanut oil, and chili powder.

2. Place the bowl in the Air Fryer and cook for 9 to 14 -minutes, until the salmon is just cooked through and firm and the vegetables are crisp-tender, stirring once. Serve instantly over hot cooked brown rice or polenta, if desired.

Nutrition:

- Calories: 116

- Fat: 3g (23% of calories from fat)

- Saturated Fat: 0g

- Protein: 18g

- Carbohydrates: 5g

- Sodium: 136mg

- Fiber: 0g

- Sugar: 3g

- 22% DV vitamin A

- 96% DV vitamin C

Scallops with Green Vegetables

Preparation Time: 15 Minutes

Cooking Time: 8 to 11 Minutes

Servings: 4

Ingredients:

- 1 cup of green beans

- 1 cup of frozen peas

- 1 cup of frozen chopped broccoli

- 2 teaspoons of olive oil

- ½ teaspoon of dried basil

- ½ teaspoon of dried oregano

- 12 ounces of sea scallops

Directions:

1. In an enormous bowl, toss the green beans, peas, and broccoli with the olive oil. Place in the Air Fryer basket. Air-fry for 4 to 6 minutes, or until the vegetables are crisp-tender.

2. Remove the vegetables from the Air Fryer basket and sprinkle with the herbs. Set aside.

3. In the Air Fryer basket, put the scallops and air-fry for 4 to 5 minutes, or until the scallops are firm and reach an internal temperature of just 145°F on a meat thermometer.

4. Toss scallops with the vegetables and serve immediately.

Nutrition:

- Calories: 124

- Fat: 3g (22% of calories from fat)

- Saturated Fat: 0g

- Protein: 14g

- Carbohydrates: 11g

- Sodium: 56mg

- Fiber: 3g

- Sugar: 3g

- 15% DV vitamin A

- 46% DV vitamin C

Cilantro Lime Shrimps

Preparation Time: 25 minutes

Cooking Time: 21 minutes

Servings: 4

Ingredients:

- 1/2-pound of shrimp, peeled, deveined

- 1/2 teaspoon of minced garlic

- 1 tablespoon of chopped cilantro

- 1/2 teaspoon of paprika

- ¾ teaspoon of salt

- 1/2 teaspoon of ground cumin

- 2 tablespoons of lemon juice

Directions:

1. Take 6 wooden skewers and let them soak in warm water for 20 minutes.

2. Meanwhile, switch on the Air Fryer, insert the fryer basket, grease it with olive oil, then shut with its lid, set the fryer at 350 ºF, and let preheat.

3. Whisk together lemon juice, paprika, salt, cumin, and garlic in a large bowl, then add shrimps and toss until well coated.

4. Drain the skewers and then thread shrimps in them.

5. Open the fryer, add shrimps in it in a single layer, spray oil over them, close with its lid and cook for 8 minutes until nicely golden and cooked, turning the skewers halfway through the frying.

6. When the Air Fryer beeps, open its lid, transfer shrimps onto a serving plate, and keep them warm.

7. Cook remaining shrimp skewers the same way and serve.

Nutrition:

- Calories: 59 Cal

- Carbs: 0.3 g

- Fat: 1.5 g

- Protein: 11 g

- Fiber: 0 g

Juicy & Healthy Meatballs

Preparation Time: 10 minutes

Cooking Time: 14 minutes

Servings: 4

Ingredients:

- 1 lb. of ground beef

- 1 tsp. of garlic powder

- 1 egg, lightly beaten

- 1/4 cup of breadcrumbs

- 1/2 onion, diced

- Pepper

- Salt

Directions:

1. Add all ingredients into the enormous bowl and mix until well combined.

2. Place the dehydrating tray in a multi-level Air Fryer basket and place the basket in the instant pot.

3. Form meatballs with the meat mixture, and place them on dehydrating tray.

4. Seal pot with Air Fryer lid and select air fry mode, then set the temperature to 390 F and timer for 14 minutes. Turn meatballs halfway through.

5. Serve and enjoy.

Nutrition:

- Calories: 261

- Fat: 8.5 g

- Carbohydrates: 6.8 g

- Sugar: 1.3 g

- Protein: 37 g

- Cholesterol: 142 mg

Feta Lemon Meatballs

Preparation Time: 10 minutes

Cooking Time: 8 minutes

Servings: 4

Ingredients:

- 5 oz. of ground beef

- 1/2 tbsp. of lemon zest, grated

- 1 tbsp. of fresh oregano, chopped

- 2 oz. of feta cheese, crumbled

- 2 tbsp. of almond flour

- Pepper

- Salt

Directions:

1. Add all ingredients into the enormous mixing bowl and mix until well combined.

2. Place the dehydrating tray in a multi-level Air Fryer basket and place the basket in the instant pot.

3. Form meatballs with the meat mixture and place them on dehydrating tray.

4. Seal pot with Air Frye- lid and select air fry mode, and then set the temperature to 400 ºF and timer for 8 minutes. Turn meatballs halfway through.

5. Serve and enjoy.

Nutrition:

- Calories: 128

- Fat: 7 g

- Carbohydrates: 2.2 g

- Sugar: 0.7 g

- Protein: 13.7 g

- Cholesterol: 44 mg

Cheesy Meatballs

Preparation Time: 10 minutes

Cooking Time: 20 minutes

Servings: 4

Ingredients:

- 1/2 lb. of ground beef

- 1/2 tsp. of garlic powder

- 1/2 tsp. of onion powder

- 1/2 lb. of Italian sausage

- 1/2 cup of Cheddar cheese, shredded

- 1/2 tsp. of black pepper

Directions:

1. Add all ingredients into the enormous mixing bowl and mix until well combined.

2. Place the dehydrating tray in a multi-level Air Fryer basket and place the basket in the instant pot.

3. Form meatballs with the meat mixture, and place them on dehydrating tray.

4. Seal pot with Air Fryer lid and select air fry mode, and then set the temperature to 370 ºF and timer for 20 minutes. Turn meatballs halfway through.

5. Serve and enjoy.

Nutrition:

- Calories: 357

- Fat: 24.3 g

- Carbohydrates: 0.8 g

- Sugar: 0.3 g

- Protein: 31.9 g

- Cholesterol: 113 mg

Honey Mustard Meatballs

Preparation Time: 10 minutes

Cooking Time: 15 minutes

Servings: 2

Ingredients:

- 5 oz. of ground pork

- 1/2 tsp. of honey

- 1/2 tsp. of garlic paste

- 1/2 tbsp. of Cheddar cheese, grated

- 1/2 tbsp. of fresh basil

- 1/2 onion, diced

- 1/2 tsp. of mustard

- Pepper

- Salt

Directions:

1. Add all ingredients into the enormous mixing bowl and mix until well combined.

2. Place the dehydrating tray in a multi-level Air Fryer basket and place the basket in the instant pot.

3. Form meatballs with the meat mixture, and place them on dehydrating tray.

4. Seal pot with Air Fryer lid and select air fry mode, and then set the temperature to 390 ℉ and timer for 15 minutes. Turn meatballs halfway through.

5. Serve and enjoy.

Nutrition:

- Calories: 130

- Fat: 3.4 g

- Carbohydrates: 4.6 g

- Sugar: 2.7 g

- Protein: 19.6 g

- Cholesterol: 54 mg

Greek Meatballs

Preparation Time: 10 minutes

Cooking Time: 20 minutes

Servings: 4

Ingredients:

- 1 lb. of ground beef

- 1 egg, lightly beaten

- 1/4 cup of parsley, chopped

- 4 oz. of feta cheese, crumbled

- 1 tbsp. of garlic, minced

- 1/4 cup of breadcrumbs

- 1/2 onion, chopped

- 1/2 lb. of ground lamb

- Pepper

- Salt

Directions:

1. Add all ingredients into the mixing bowl and mix until well combined.

2. Place the dehydrating tray in a multi-level Air Fryer basket and place the basket in the instant pot.

   Form meatballs with the meat mixture, and place them on dehydrating tray.

3. Seal the pot with Air Fryer lid and select back mode, and then set the temperature to 380 ºF and timer for 25 minutes. Turn meatballs halfway through.

4. Serve and enjoy.

Nutrition:

- Calories: 443

- Fat: 18.8 g

- Carbohydrates: 8.3 g

- Sugar: 2.3 g

- Protein: 57 g

- Cholesterol: 219 mg

Steak Burgers

Preparation Time: 10 minutes

Cooking Time: 12 minutes

Servings: 4

Ingredients:

- 1 lb. of ground beef

- 1/8 tsp. of cayenne pepper

- 2 tsp. of paprika

- 2 tsp. of mustard powder

- 1 tsp. of Worcestershire sauce

- 1 tsp. of tomato paste

- 3 garlic cloves, minced

- 1/2 small onion, minced

- Pepper

- Salt

Directions:

1. Add all ingredients into the enormous bowl and mix until well combined.

2. Place the dehydrating tray in a multi-level Air Fryer basket and place the basket in the instant pot.

3. Make small patties from the meat mixture and place them on dehydrating tray.

4. Seal pot with Air Fryer lid and select air fry mode, then set the temperature to 320 ºF and timer for 12 minutes. Turn patties halfway through.

5. Serve and enjoy.

Nutrition:

- Calories: 231

- Fat: 7.7 g

- Carbohydrates: 3.3 g

- Sugar: 1 g

- Protein: 35.3 g

- Cholesterol: 101 mg

Juicy Lamb Chops

Preparation Time: 10 minutes

Cooking Time: 14 minutes

Servings: 4

Ingredients:

- 4 lamb chops

- 2 garlic cloves, minced

- 2 tbsp. of olive oil

- Pepper

- Salt

Directions:

1. Coat lamb chops with oil and rubs with garlic, pepper, and salt.

2. Place the dehydrating tray in a multi-level Air Fryer basket and place the basket in the instant pot.

3. Place lamb chops on dehydrating tray.

4. Seal pot with Air Fryer lid and select air fry mode, then set the temperature to 350 ºF and timer for 14 minutes. Turn lamb chops halfway through.

5. Serve and enjoy.

Nutrition:

- Calories: 313

- Fat: 16.9 g

- Carbohydrates: 0.5 g

- Sugar: 0 g

- Protein: 38 g

- Cholesterol: 122 mg

Lamb Roast

Preparation Time: 10 minutes

Cooking Time: 15 minutes

Servings: 2

Ingredients:

- 10 oz. of lamb leg roast

- 1 tsp. of dried thyme

- 1 tsp. of dried rosemary

- 1 tbsp. of olive oil

- Pepper

- Salt

Directions:

1. Coat lamb roast with olive oil and rub with thyme, rosemary, pepper, and salt.

2. Place the dehydrating tray in a multi-level Air Fryer basket and place the basket in the instant pot.

3. Place lamb roast on dehydrating tray.

4. Seal pot with Air Fryer lid and select air fry mode, then set the temperature to 360 F and timer for 15 minutes.

5. Serve and enjoy.

Nutrition:

- Calories: 319

- Fat: 16.6 g

- Carbohydrates: 0.7 g

- Sugar: 0 g

- Protein: 40 g

- Cholesterol: 123 mg

Chicken in Tomato Juice

Preparation Time: 20 Minutes

Cooking Time: 15 Minutes

Servings: 3

Ingredients:

- 350 g of chicken fillet

- 200 g of tomato juice

- 100 g of tomatoes

- 2 teaspoon of basil

- 1 teaspoon of chili

- 1 teaspoon of oregano

- 1 teaspoon of rosemary

- 1 teaspoon of olive oil

- 1 teaspoon of mint

- 1 teaspoon of lemon juice

Directions:

1. Take a bowl and make the tomato sauce: combine basil, chili, oregano, rosemary, and olive oil, mint, and lemon juice and stir the mixture very carefully.

2. You can use a hand mixer to mix the mass. It will make the mixture smooth.

3. Take a chicken fillet and separate it into 3 pieces.

4. Put the meat into the tomato mixture and leave for 15 minutes.

5. Meanwhile, preheat the Air Fryer oven to 230 ºC.

6. Put the meat mixture on the tray and put it in the oven for at least 15 minutes.

Nutrition:

- Calories: 258 kcal

- Proteins: 34.8 grams

- Fats: 10.5 grams

- Carbohydrates: 5.0 grams

Salmon on Bed of Fennel and Carrot

Preparation Time: 15 Minutes

Cooking Time: 13 to 14 Minutes

Servings: 2

Ingredients:

- 1 fennel bulb, thinly sliced

- 1 large carrot, peeled and sliced

- 1 small onion, thinly sliced

- ¼ cup of low-fat sour cream

- ¼ teaspoon of coarsely ground pepper

- 2 (5 ounces) of salmon fillets

Directions:

1. Combine the fennel, carrot, and onion in a bowl and toss.

2. Put the vegetable mixture into a 6-inch metal pan. Roast in the Air Fryer for 4 minutes or until the vegetables are crisp-tender.

3. Remove the pan from the Air Fryer. Stir in the sour cream and sprinkle the vegetables with the pepper.

4. Top with the salmon fillets.

5. Return the pan to the Air Fryer. Roast for another 9 to 10 minutes or until the salmon just barely flakes when tested with a fork.

Nutrition:

- Calories: 253

- Fat: 9g (32% calories from fat)

- Saturated Fat: 1g

- Protein: 31g

- Carbohydrates: 12g

- Sodium: 115mg

- Fiber 3g

- Sugar: 5g

- 130% DV vitamin A

- 15% DV vitamin C

Roasted Vegetable Chicken Salad

Preparation Time: 10 Minutes

Cooking Time: 10 to 13 Minutes

Servings: 4

Ingredients:

- 3 (4-ounce) of low-sodium boneless skinless chicken breasts, cut into 1-inch cubes (see Tip)

- 1 small red onion, sliced

- 1 red bell pepper, sliced

- 1 cup green beans, cut into 1-inch pieces

- 2 tablespoons of low-fat ranch salad dressing

- 2 tablespoons of freshly squeezed lemon juice

- ½ teaspoon of dried basil

- 4 cups of mixed lettuce

Directions:

1. In the Air Fryer basket, roast the chicken, red onion, red bell pepper, and green beans for 10 to 13 minutes, or until the chicken reaches an internal temperature of 165 °F on a meat thermometer, tossing the food in the basket once during cooking.

2. While the chicken cooks, in a serving bowl, mix the ranch dressing, lemon juice, and basil.

3. Transfer the chicken and vegetables to a serving bowl and toss with the dressing to coat. Serve immediately on lettuce leaves.

Nutrition:

- Calories: 113

- Fat: 1g (8% of calories from fat)

- Saturated Fat: 0g

- Protein: 19g

- Carbohydrates: 7g

- Sodium: 138g

- Fiber: 2g

- Sugar: 3g

- 13% DV vitamin A

- 42% DV vitamin C

Warm Chicken and Spinach Salad

Preparation Time: 10 Minutes

Cooking Time: 16 to 20 Minutes

Servings: 4

Ingredients:

- 3 (5-ounce) of low-sodium boneless skinless chicken breasts, cut into 1-inch cubes

- 5 teaspoons of olive oil

- ½ teaspoon of dried thyme

- 1 medium red onion, sliced

- 1 red bell pepper, sliced

- 1 small zucchini, cut into strips

- 3 tablespoons of freshly squeezed lemon juice

- 6 cups of fresh baby spinach

Directions:

1. In a large bowl, mix the chicken with olive oil and thyme. Toss to coat. Transfer to a medium metal bowl and roast for 8 minutes in the Air Fryer.

2. Add the red onion, red bell pepper, and zucchini. Roast for 8 to 12 minutes more, stirring once during cooking, or until the chicken reaches an internal temperature of 165 °F on a meat thermometer.

3. Remove the bowl from the Air Fryer and stir in the lemon juice.

4. Put the spinach in a serving bowl and top with the chicken mixture. Toss to combine and serve immediately.

Nutrition:

- Calories: 214

- Fat: 7g (29% of calories from fat)

- Saturated Fat: 1g

- Protein: 28g

- Carbohydrates: 7g

- Sodium: 116mg

- Fiber: 2g

- Sugar: 4g

- 90% DV vitamin A

- 69% DV vitamin C

Nutty Chicken Nuggets

Preparation Time: 10 Minutes

Cooking Time: 10 to 13 Minutes

Servings: 4

Ingredients:

- 1 egg white

- 1 tablespoon of freshly squeezed lemon juice

- ½ teaspoon of dried basil

- ½ teaspoon of ground paprika

- 1 pound of low-sodium boneless skinless chicken breasts, cut into 1½-inch cubes

- ½ cup of ground almonds

- 2 slices of low-sodium whole-wheat bread, crumbled

Directions:

1. In a shallow bowl, beat the egg white, lemon juice, basil, and paprika with a fork until foamy.

2. Add the chicken and stir to coat.

3. On a plate, mix the almonds and bread crumbs.

4. Toss the chicken cubes in the almond and bread crumb mixture until coated.

5. Bake the nuggets in the Air Fryer, in two batches, for 10 to 13 minutes, or until the chicken reaches an internal temperature of 165 °F on a meat thermometer. Serve immediately.

Nutrition:

- Calories: 249

- Fat: 8g (29% of calories from fat)

- Saturated Fat: 1g

- Protein: 32g

- Carbohydrates: 13g

- Sodium: 137mg

- Fiber: 3g

- Sugar: 3g

- 3% DV vitamin A

- 2% DV vitamin C

Spicy Chicken Meatballs

Preparation Time: 10 Minutes

Cooking Time: 11 to 14 Minutes

Servings: 24

Ingredients:

- 1 medium red onion, minced

- 2 garlic cloves, minced

- 1 jalapeño pepper, minced

- 2 teaspoons of olive oil

- 3 tablespoons of ground almonds

- 1 egg

- 1 teaspoon of dried thyme

- 1 pound of ground chicken breast

Directions:

1. In a 6-by-2-inch pan, combine the red onion, garlic, jalapeño, and olive oil. Bake for 3 to 4 minutes in the Air Fryer, or until the vegetables are crisp-tender. Transfer to a medium bowl.

2. Mix in the almonds, egg, and thyme to the vegetable mixture. Add the chicken and mix until just combined.

3. Form the chicken mixture into about 24 (1-inch) balls. Bake the meatballs, in batches, for 8 to 10 minutes, until the chicken reaches an internal temperature of 165 °F on a meat thermometer.

Nutrition:

- Calories: 185

- Fat: 7g (34% of calories from fat)

- Saturated Fat: 1g

- Protein: 29g

- Carbohydrates: 5g

- Sodium: 55mg

- Fiber: 1g

- Sugar: 3g

- 2% DV vitamin A

- 10% DV vitamin C

Chicken Wings with Curry

Preparation Time: 15 Minutes

Cooking Time: 20 Minutes

Servings: 4

Ingredients:

- 400 g chicken wings

- 30 g curry

- 1 teaspoon of chili

- 1 teaspoon of cayenne pepper

- 1 teaspoon of salt

- 1 lemon

- 1 teaspoon of basil

- 1 teaspoon of oregano

- 3 teaspoon of mustard

- 1 teaspoon of olive oil

Directions:

1. Rub the wings with chili, curry, cayenne pepper, salt, basil, and oregano.

2. Put it in the bowl and mix it very carefully.

3. Leave the mixture at least for 10 minutes in the fridge.

4. Remove the mixture from the fridge and add mustard and sprinkle with chopped lemon. Stir the mixture gently again.

5. Spray the pan with olive oil and put the wings in it.

6. Preheat the Air Fryer oven to 180 ºC and put wings there.

7. Cook it for 20 minutes.

Nutrition:

- Calories: 244 kcal

- Proteins: 30.8 grams

- Fats: 10.6 grams

- Carbohydrates: 7.2 grams

Stuffed Chicken

Preparation Time: 15 Minutes

Cooking Time: 30 Minutes

Servings: 4

Ingredients:

- 2 chicken breasts

- 2 tomatoes

- 200 g basil

- 1 teaspoon of black pepper

- 1 teaspoon of cayenne pepper

- 100 g of tomato juice

- 40 g of goat cheese

Directions:

1. Make a "pocket" from the chicken breasts and rub it with black pepper and cayenne pepper.

2. Slice tomatoes and chop basil.

3. Chop the goat cheese.

4. Combine all the ingredients together—it will be the filling for breasts.

5. Fill the chicken breasts with this mixture.

6. Take a needle, thread, and sew "pockets."

7. Preheat the Air Fryer oven to 200 ºC. Place the chicken breasts in the tray and pour it with tomato juice.

8. Serve.

Nutrition:

- Calories: 312 kcal

- Proteins: 41.6 grams

- Fats: 13.4 grams

- Carbohydrates: 5.6 grams

Mesquite Pork Chops

Preparation Time: 10 minutes

Cooking Time: 14 minutes

Servings: 2

Ingredients:

- 2 pork chops

- 1 tbsp. of olive oil

- 2 tbsp. of honey

- 1 1/2 tbsp. of mesquite seasoning Pepper

- Salt

Directions:

1. Mix together oil, honey, mesquite seasoning, pepper, salt and rub all over pork chops.

2. Place the dehydrating tray in a multi-level Air Fryer basket and place the basket in the instant pot.

3. Place pork chops on dehydrating tray.

4. Seal pot with Air Fryer lid and select air fry mode, then set the temperature to 380 ºF and timer for 14 minutes. Turn pork chops halfway through.

5. Serve and enjoy.

Nutrition:

- Calories: 390

- Fat: 27.1 g

- Carbohydrates: 19.1 g

- Sugar: 17.3 g

- Protein: 18.4 g

- Cholesterol: 69 mg

Ranch Pork Chops

Preparation Time: 10 minutes

Cooking Time: 12 minutes

Servings: 4

Ingredients:

- 4 pork chops

- 1 egg, lightly beaten

- 1 packet of ranch seasoning 2 cups breadcrumbs

- 1/2 cup of milk

- Pepper

- Salt

Directions:

1. In a shallow bowl, whisk egg, milk, pepper, and salt.

2. In a shallow dish, mix together breadcrumbs and ranch seasoning.

3. Dip pork chops in egg and coat with breadcrumbs.

4. Place the dehydrating tray in a multi-level Air Fryer basket and place basket in the instant pot.

5. Place pork chops on dehydrating tray.

6. Seal pot with Air Fryer lid and select air fry mode then set the temperature to 360 ºF and timer for 12 minutes. Turn pork chops halfway through.

7. Serve and enjoy.

Nutrition:

- Calories: 522

- Fat: 24.5 g

- Carbohydrates: 40.5 g

- Sugar: 4.8 g

- Protein: 27.6 g

- Cholesterol: 112 mg

Pork Chops with Peanut Sauce

Preparation Time: 20 minutes

Cooking Time: 12 minutes

Servings: 4

Ingredients:

For Chops:

- 1 teaspoon of fresh ginger, minced

- 1 garlic clove, minced

- 2 tablespoons of soy sauce

- 1 tablespoon of olive oil

- 1 teaspoon of hot pepper sauce

- 1-pound of boneless pork chop, cubed into 1-inch size

For Peanut Sauce:

- 1 tablespoon of olive oil

- 1 shallot, finely chopped

- 1 garlic clove, minced

- 1 teaspoon of ground coriander

- ¾ cup of ground peanuts

- 1 teaspoon of hot pepper sauce

- ¾ cup of coconut milk

Directions:

1. For the pork: in a bowl, mix together the ginger, garlic, soy sauce, oil, and hot pepper sauce.

2. Add the pork chops and generously coat with mixture.

3. Place at the room temperature for about 15 minutes.

4. Set the temperature of Air Fryer to 390 ºF. Grease an Air Fryer basket.

5. Arrange chops into the prepared Air Fryer basket in a single layer.

6. Air fry for about 12 minutes.

7. Meanwhile, for the sauce: in a pan, heat oil over medium heat and sauté the shallot and garlic for about 2-3 minutes.

8. Add the coriander and sauté for about 1 minute.

9. Stir in the remaining ingredients and cook for about 5 minutes, stirring continuously.

10.   Remove the pan of sauce from heat and let it cool slightly.

11.   Remove the chops from Air Fryer and transfer onto serving plates.

12.   Serve immediately with the topping of peanut sauce.

Nutrition:

- Calories: 725

- Carbohydrates: 9.5g

- Protein: 34.4g

- Fat: 62.9g

- Sugar: 2.8g

- Sodium: 543mg

Pork Spare Ribs

Preparation Time: 15 minutes

Cooking Time: 20 minutes

Servings: 6

Ingredients:

- 5-6 garlic cloves, minced

- ½ cup of rice vinegar

- 2 tablespoons of soy sauce

- Salt and ground black pepper, as required

- 12: 1-inch pork spare ribs

- ½ cup of cornstarch

- 2 tablespoons of olive oil

Directions:

1. In an enormous bowl, mix the garlic, vinegar, soy sauce, salt, and black pepper.

2. Add the ribs and generously coat with mixture.

3. Refrigerate to marinate overnight.

4. In a shallow bowl, place the cornstarch.

5. Coat the ribs evenly with cornstarch and then, drizzle with oil.

6. Set the temperature of Air Fryer to 390 °F. Grease an Air Fryer basket.

7. Arrange ribs into the prepared Air Fryer basket in a single layer.

8. Air fry for about 10 minutes per side.

9. Remove from Air Fryer and transfer the ribs onto serving plates.

10.   Serve immediately.

Nutrition:

- Calories: 557

- Carbohydrate: 11g

- Protein: 35g

- Fat: 51.3g

- Sugar: 0.1g

- Sodium: 997mg

BBQ Pork Ribs

Preparation Time: 15 minutes

Cooking Time: 26 minutes

Servings: 4

Ingredients:

- ¼ cup of honey, divided

- ¾ cup of BBQ sauce

- 2 tablespoons of tomato ketchup

- 1 tablespoon of Worcestershire sauce*

- 1 tablespoon of soy sauce

- ½ teaspoon of garlic powder

- Freshly ground white pepper to taste

- 1¾ pounds of pork ribs

Directions:

1. In a basin, mix 3 tablespoons of honey and the remaining ingredients except for pork ribs.

2. Add the pork ribs and generously coat with the mixture.

3. Refrigerate to marinate for about 20 minutes.

4. Set the temperature of Air Fryer to 355 ºF. Grease an Air Fryer basket.

5. Arrange ribs into the prepared Air Fryer basket in a single layer.

6. Air fry for about 13 minutes per side.

7. Remove from Air Fryer and transfer the ribs onto plates.

8. Drizzle with the remaining honey and serve immediately.

9. (Note - Worcestershire sauce* - The other ingredients that make up this savory sauce usually include onions, molasses, high fructose corn syrup: depending on the country of production), salt, garlic, tamarind, cloves, chili pepper extract, water and natural flavorings.

Nutrition:

- Calories: 691

- Carbohydrates: 37.7g

- Protein: 53.1g

- Fat: 31.3g

- Sugar: 32.2g

- Sodium: 991mg

Glazed Pork Shoulder

Preparation Time: 15 minutes

Cooking Time: 18 minutes

Servings: 5

Ingredients:

- 1/3 cup of soy sauce

- 2 tablespoons of sugar

- 1 tablespoon of honey

- 2 pounds of pork shoulder, cut into 1½-inch thick slices

Directions:

1. In a bowl, mix together all the soy sauce, sugar, and honey.

2. Add the pork and generously coat with marinade.

3. Cover and refrigerate to marinate for about 4-6 hours.

4. Set the temperature of Air Fryer to 335 ℉. Grease an Air Fryer basket.

5. Place the pork shoulder into the prepared Air Fryer basket.

6. Air fry for about 10 minutes and then, another 6-8 minutes at 390 ℉.

7. Remove from Air Fryer and transfer the pork shoulder onto a platter.

8. With a piece of foil, cover the pork for about 10 minutes before serving.

9. Enjoy!

Nutrition:

- Calories: 475

- Carbohydrates: 8g

- Protein: 36.1g

- Fat: 32.4g

- Sugar: 7.1g

- Sodium: 165mg

Pork Shoulder with Pineapple Sauce

Preparation Time: 20 minutes

Cooking Time: 24 minutes

Servings: 3

Ingredients:

For Pork:

- 10½ ounces of pork shoulder, cut into bite-sized pieces

- 2 pinches of Maggi seasoning

- 1 teaspoon of light soy sauce

- Dash of sesame oil

- 1 egg

- ¼ cup of plain flour

For Sauce:

- 1 teaspoon of olive oil

- 1 medium of onion, sliced

- 1 tablespoon of garlic, minced

- 1 large pineapple slice, cubed

- 1 medium tomato, chopped

- 2 tablespoons of tomato sauce

- 2 tablespoons of oyster sauce

- 1 tablespoon of Worcestershire sauce

- 1 teaspoon of sugar

- 1 tablespoon of water

- ½ tablespoon of corn flour

Directions:

1 For the pork: in a large bowl, mix together the Maggi seasoning, soy sauce, and sesame oil.

2 Add the pork cubes and generously mix with the mixture.

3 Refrigerate to marinate for about 4-6 hours.

4 In a shallow dish, beat the egg.

5 In another dish, place the plain flour.

6 Dip the cubed pork in beaten egg and then, coat evenly with the flour.

7 Set the temperature of Air Fryer to 248°F. Grease an Air Fryer basket.

8 Arrange pork cubes into the prepared Air Fryer basket in a single layer.

9 Air fry for about 20 minutes.

10 Meanwhile, for the sauce: in a skillet, heat oil over medium heat and sauté the onion and garlic for about 1 minute.

11 Add the pineapple and tomato and cook for about 1 minute.

12 Add the tomato sauce, oyster sauce, Worcestershire sauce, and sugar and stir to combine.

13 Meanwhile, in a bowl, mix together the water and the corn flour.

14 Add the corn flour mixture into the sauce, stirring continuously.

15 Cook until the sauce is thickened enough, stirring continuously.

16 Remove pork cubes from Air Fryer and add into the sauce.

17 Cook for about 1-2 minutes or until coated completely.

18 Remove from the heat and serve hot.

(Note: if you don't have fresh pineapple in hands, then you can use canned pineapple. But remember to skip sugar from the sauce).

Nutrition:

- Calories: 557

- Carbohydrates: 57.5g

- Protein: 28.8g

- Fat: 25.1g

- Sugar: 35.1g

- Sodium: 544mg

Bacon Wrapped Pork Tenderloin

Preparation Time: 15 minutes

Cooking Time: 30 minutes

Servings: 4

Ingredients:

- 1: 1½ pound of pork tenderloins

- 4 bacon strips

- 2 tablespoons of Dijon mustard

Directions:

1. Coat the tenderloin evenly with mustard.

2. Wrap the tenderloin with bacon strips.

3. Set the temperature of Air Fryer to 360°F. Grease an Air Fryer basket.

4. Arrange pork tenderloin into the prepared Air Fryer basket.

5. Air fry for about 15 minutes.

6. Flip and air fry for another 10-15 minutes.

7. Remove from Air Fryer and transfer the pork tenderloin onto a platter, wait for about 5 minutes before slicing.

8. Cut the tenderloin into desired size slices and serve.

Nutrition:

- Calories: 504

- Carbohydrates: 0.8g

- Protein: 61.9

- Fat: 26.2g

- Sugar: 9.1g

- Sodium: 867mg

Pork Tenderloin with Bell Peppers

Preparation Time: 20 minutes

Cooking Time: 15 minutes

Servings: 3

Ingredients:

- 1 big red bell pepper, seeded and cut into thin strips

- 1 red onion, thinly sliced

- 2 teaspoons of Herbs de Provence

- Salt and ground black pepper, as required

- 1 tablespoon of olive oil

- 10½-ounces of pork tenderloin, cut into 4 pieces

- ½ tablespoon of Dijon mustard

Directions:

1. In a bowl, add the bell pepper, onion, Herbs de Provence, salt, black pepper, and ½ tablespoon of oil and toss to coat well.

2. Rub the pork pieces with mustard, salt, and black pepper.

3. Drizzle with the remaining oil.

4. Set the temperature of Air Fryer to 390°F. Grease an Air Fryer pan.

5. Place bell pepper mixture into the prepared Air Fryer pan and top with the pork pieces.

6. Air fry for about 15 minutes, flipping once halfway through.

7. Remove from Air Fryer and transfer the pork mixture onto serving plates.

8. Serve hot.

Nutrition:

- Calories: 218

- Carbohydrates: 7.1g

- Protein: 27.7g

- Fat: 8.8g

- Sugar: 3.7g

- Sodium: 110mg

Pork Tenderloin with Bacon & Veggies

Preparation Time: 20 minutes

Cooking Time: 28 minutes

Servings: 3

Ingredients:

- 3 potatoes

- ¾ pound of frozen green beans

- 6 bacon slices

- 3: 6-ounces of pork tenderloins

- 2 tablespoons of olive oil

Directions:

1 Set the temperature of Air Fryer to 390°F. Grease an Air Fryer basket.

2 With a fork, pierce the potatoes.

3 Place potatoes into the prepared Air Fryer basket and air fry for about 15 minutes.

4 Wrap one bacon slice around 4-6 green beans.

5 Coat the pork tenderloins with oil

6 After 15 minutes, add the pork tenderloins into Air Fryer basket with potatoes and air fry for about 5-6 minutes.

7 Remove the pork tenderloins from the basket.

8 Place bean rolls into the basket and top with the pork tenderloins.

9 Air fry for another 7 minutes.

10 Remove from the Air Fryer and transfer the pork tenderloins onto a platter.

11 Cut each tenderloin into desired size slices.

12 Serve alongside the potatoes and green beans rolls.

Nutrition:

- Calories: 918

- Carbohydrates: 42.4g

- Protein: 77.9g

- Fat: 47.7g

- Sugar: 4g

- Sodium: 1400mg

Pork Loin with Potatoes

Preparation Time: 15 minutes

Cooking Time: 25 minutes

Servings: 5

Ingredients:

- 2 pounds of pork loin

- 3 tablespoons of olive oil, divided

- 1 teaspoon of fresh parsley, chopped

- Salt and ground black pepper, as required

- 3 large red potatoes, chopped

- ½ teaspoon of garlic powder

- ½ teaspoon of red pepper flakes, crushed

Directions:

1. Coat the pork loin with oil and then season evenly with parsley, salt, and black pepper.

2. In an enormous bowl, mix the potatoes, remaining oil, garlic powder, red pepper flakes, salt, and black pepper and toss to coat well.

3. Set the temperature of Air Fryer to 325°F. Grease an Air Fryer basket.

4. Place loin into the prepared Air Fryer basket.

5. Arrange potato pieces around the pork loin.

6. Air fry for about 25 minutes.

7. Remove from Air Fryer and transfer the pork loin onto a platter, wait for about 5 minutes before slicing.

8. Cut the pork loin into desired size slices and serve alongside the potatoes.

Nutrition:

- Calories: 556

- Carbohydrates: 29.6g

- Protein: 44.9g

- Fat: 28.3g

- Sugar: 1.9g

- Sodium: 132mg

Sugar Stuffed Bell Peppers

Preparation Time: 10-20 minutes

Cooking Time: 30 minutes

Servings: 4

Ingredients:

- 1 lb. of turkey meat, ground.

- 5 oz. of canned green chilies; chopped.

- 1 cup of water

- 1 jalapeno pepper; chopped.

- 2 tsp. of chili powder

- 1 tsp. of garlic powder

- 1 tsp. of cumin, ground.

- 2 green onions; chopped.

- 1 avocado; chopped

- Salt to the taste

- 1/2 cup of whole wheat panko

- 4 bell peppers, tops, and seeds discarded

- 4 pepper jack cheese slices

- Crushed tortilla chips

- Pico de Gallo

For the chipotle sauce:

- Zest from 1 lime

- Juice from 1 lime

- 1/2 cup of sour cream

- 2 tbsp. of chipotle in adobo sauce

- 1/8 tsp. of garlic powder

Directions:

1. In a bowl, mix sour cream with chipotle in adobo sauce, lime zest and lime juice and garlic powder, stir well and keep in the fridge until you serve it.

2. In a bowl, mix turkey meat with green onions, green chilies, breadcrumbs, jalapeno, cumin, salt, chili powder and garlic powder, stir very well and stuff your peppers with this mix.

3. Add 1 cup water to your instant pot, add peppers in the steamer basket, close the lid and cook at High for 15 minutes.

4. Release the pressure naturally for 10 minutes, then release the remaining pressure by turning the valve to 'Venting,' transfer bell peppers to a pan, add

cheese on top, introduce in preheated broiler and broil until cheese is browned.

5. Divide bell peppers or plates, top with the chipotle sauce you've made earlier and serve.

Nutrition:

- Calories: 220

- Fat: 11g

- Protein: 5g

- Sugar: 2g

- Carbohydrates: 13g

- Fiber: 4g

- Sodium: 325mg

- Cholesterol: 67mg

Chapter 4. Vegetable and Potatoes Recipes

Eggplant Surprise

Preparation Time: 10-20 minutes

Cooking Time: 17 minutes

Servings: 4

Ingredients:

- 1 eggplant, roughly chopped

- 3 zucchinis, roughly chopped

- 3 tbsp. of extra virgin olive oil

- 3 tomatoes, sliced

- 2 tbsp. of lemon juice

- 1 tsp. of thyme; dried

- 1 tsp. of oregano; dried

- Salt and black pepper to the taste

Directions:

1. Put eggplant pieces in your instant pot.

2. Add zucchinis and tomatoes.

3. In a bowl, mix lemon juice with salt, pepper, thyme, oregano and oil and stir well.

4. Pour this over veggies, toss to coat, seal the instant pot lid and cook at High for 7 minutes.

5. Quick-release the pressure, carefully open the lid; divide among plates and serve.

Nutrition:
*   Calories: 160
*   Fat: 7g
*   Protein: 1g
*   Sugar: 6g
*   Carbohydrates: 19g
*   Fiber: 8g
*   Sodium: 20mg

Carrots and Turnips

Preparation Time: 10-20 minutes

Cooking Time: 15 minutes

Servings: 4

Ingredients:

- 2 turnips, peeled and sliced

- 1 small onion; chopped.

- 1 tsp. of lemon juice

- 1 tsp. of cumin, ground.

- 3 carrots, sliced

- 1 tbsp. of extra-virgin olive oil

- 1 cup of water

- Salt and black pepper to the taste

Directions:

1. Set your instant pot on Sauté mode; add oil and heat it up.

2. Add onion, stir and sauté for 2 minutes.

3. Add turnips, carrots, cumin and lemon juice, stir and cook for 1 minute.

4. Add salt, pepper, and water; then stir well. Close the lid and cook at High for 6 minutes.

5. Quickly release the pressure, open the instant pot lid, and divide turnips and carrots among plates and serve.

Nutrition:

- Calories: 170
- Fat: 9g
- Protein: 1g
- Sugar: 5g
- Carbohydrates: 19g
- Fiber: 7g
- Sodium: 475mg

Shrimp and Asparagus

Preparation Time: 10-20 minutes

Cooking Time: 8 minutes

Servings: 4

Ingredients:

- 1 lb. of shrimp, peeled and deveined

- 1 cup of water

- 1/2 tbsp. of Cajun seasoning

- 1 tsp. of extra virgin olive oil

- 1 bunch of asparagus, trimmed

Directions:

1. Pour the water in your instant pot.

2. Put asparagus in the steamer basket of the pot and add shrimp on top.

3. Drizzle olive oil, sprinkle Cajun seasoning; and then stir well. Close the lid and cook on Low for 2 minutes.

4. Release the pressure naturally, transfer asparagus and shrimp to plates and serve.

Nutrition:

- Calories: 200

- Fat: 3g

- Protein: 8g

- Sugar: 3g

Instant Brussels Sprouts with Parmesan

Preparation Time: 10-20 minutes

Cooking Time: 16 minutes

Servings: 4

Ingredients:

- 1 lb. of Brussels sprouts, washed

- 1 cup of water

- 3 tbsp. of Parmesan, grated

- Juice of 1 lemon

- 2 tbsp. of butter

- Salt and black pepper to the taste

Directions:

1. Put sprouts in your instant pot, add salt, pepper and water; and then stir well. Close the lid and cook at High for 3 minutes.

2. Quick-release the pressure, transfer sprouts to a bowl, discard water and clean your pot.

3. Set your pot on Sauté mode; add butter and melt it.

4. Add lemon juice and stir well.

5. Add sprouts, stir and transfer to plates.

6. Add more salt, pepper if needed, and Parmesan cheese on top.

Nutrition:

- Calories: 230

- Fat: 10g

- Protein: 8g

- Sugar: 5g

Braised Fennel

Preparation Time: 10-20 minutes

Cooking Time: 22 minutes

Servings: 4

Ingredients:

- 2 fennel bulbs, trimmed and cut into quarters

- 3 tbsp. extra virgin olive oil

- 1/4 cup of white wine

- 1/4 cup of Parmesan, grated

- 3/4 cup of veggie stock

- Juice of 1/2 lemon

- 1 garlic clove; chopped.

- 1 dried red pepper

- Salt and black pepper to the taste

Directions:

1. Set your instant pot on Sauté mode; add oil and heat it up.

2. Add garlic and red pepper; then stir well. Cook for 2 minutes and discard garlic.

3. Add fennel, stir and brown it for 8 minutes.

4. Add salt, pepper, stock, wine, close the lid and cook at High for 4 minutes.

5. Quickly release the pressure, open the instant pot lid, add lemon juice, more salt and pepper if needed, and cheese.

6. Mix to coat, divide among plates and serve.

Nutrition:

- Calories: 230

- Fat: 4g

- Protein: 1g

- Sugar: 3g

Brussels Sprouts & Potatoes Dish

Preparation Time: 10-20 minutes

Cooking Time: 15 minutes

Servings: 4

Ingredients:

- 1 ½ lb. of Brussels sprouts, washed and trimmed

- 1 ½ tbsp. of bread crumbs

- 1/2 cup of beef stock

- 1 cup of new potatoes; chopped.

- 1 ½ tbsp. of butter

- Salt and black pepper to the taste

Directions:

1. Put sprouts and potatoes in your instant pot

2. Add stock, salt and pepper, close the lid and cook at High for 5 minutes.

3. Quickly release the pressure, carefully open the lid; set on Sauté mode; add butter and bread crumbs, toss to coat well, divide among plates and serve.

Nutrition:

- Calories: 150

- Fat: 8g

- Protein: 1g

- Sugar: 2g

Beet and Orange Salad

Preparation Time: 10-20 minutes

Cooking Time: 20 minutes

Servings: 4

Ingredients:

- 1 ½ lb. of beets

- 3 strips orange peel

- 2 tbsp. of cider vinegar

- 1/2 cup of orange juice

- 2 tsp. of orange zest, grated

- 2 tbsp. of brown sugar

- 2 scallions; chopped

- 2 tsp. of mustard

- 2 cups of arugula and mustard greens

Directions:

1. Scrub beets well, cut them in halves and put them in a bowl.

2. In your instant pot, mix orange peel strips with vinegar and orange juice and stir.

3. Add beets, seal the instant pot lid, cook at High for 7 minutes, and naturally release the pressure.

4. Carefully open the lid, take beets and transfer them to a bowl.

5. Discard peel strips from the pot, add mustard and sugar and stir well.

6. Add scallions, grated orange zest to beets, and toss them.

7. Add liquid from the pot over beets, toss to coat and serve on plates on top of mixed salad greens.

Nutrition:

- Calories: 164

- Fat: 5g

- Protein: 2g

- Sugar: 5g

Endives Dish

Preparation Time: 10-20 minutes

Cooking Time: 30 minutes

Servings: 4

Ingredients:

- 4 endives, trimmed

- 2 tbsp. of butter

- 1 tbsp. of white flour

- 4 slices ham

- 1/2 tsp. of nutmeg

- 14 oz. of milk

- Salt and black pepper to taste

Directions:

1. Put the endives in the steamer basket of your instant pot, add some water to the pot, cover and cook at High for 10 minutes.

2. Meanwhile, heat up a pan with the butter over medium heat, stir and melt it.

3. Add flour, stir well and cook for 3 minutes.

4. Add milk, salt, pepper and nutmeg, stir well, reduce heat to low and cook for 10 minutes.

5. Release the pressure from the pot, uncover it, transfer them to a cutting board and roll each in a slice of ham.

6. Arrange endives in a pan, add the milk mixture over them, introduce in preheated broiler and broil for 10 minutes. Slice, arrange on plates and serve.

Nutrition:

- Calories: 175

- Fat: 8g

- Protein: 1g

- Sugar: 2g

Roasted Potatoes

Preparation Time: 10-20 minutes

Cooking Time: 30 minutes

Servings: 4

Ingredients:

- 2 lb. of baby potatoes

- 5 tbsp. of vegetable oil

- 1/2 cup of stock

- 1 rosemary spring

- 5 garlic cloves

- Salt and black pepper to the taste

Directions:

1. Set your instant pot on Sauté mode; add oil and heat it up.

2. Add potatoes, rosemary and garlic, stir and brown them for 10 minutes.

3. Prick each potato with a knife, add the stock, salt and pepper to the pot, Seal the Instant Pot lid and cook at High for 7 minutes.

4. Quickly release the pressure, open the instant pot lid, divide potatoes among plates and serve.

Nutrition:

- Calories: 250

- Fat: 15g

- Protein: 2g

- Sugar: 1g

Cabbage Wedges

Preparation Time: 10 minutes

Cooking Time: 29 minutes

Servings: 6

Ingredients:

- 1 small head of green cabbage

- 6 strips of bacon, thick-cut, pastured

- 1 teaspoon of onion powder

- ½ teaspoon of ground black pepper

- 1 teaspoon of garlic powder

- ¾ teaspoon of salt

- 1/4 teaspoon of red chili flakes

- 1/2 teaspoon of fennel seeds

- 3 tablespoons of olive oil

Directions:

1. Switch on the Air Fryer, insert fryer basket, grease it with olive oil, then shut with its lid, set the fryer to 350°F, and preheat for 5 minutes.

2. Open the fryer, add bacon strips in it, close with its lid and cook for 10 minutes until nicely golden and crispy, turning the bacon halfway through the frying.

3. Meanwhile, prepare the cabbage, remove the cabbage's outer leaves, and then cut it into eight wedges, keeping the core intact.

4. Prepare the spice mix and for this, place onion powder in a bowl, add black pepper, garlic powder, salt, red chili, and fennel and stir until mixed.

5. Drizzle cabbage wedges with oil and then sprinkle with spice mix until well coated.

6. When the Air Fryer beeps, open its lid, transfer bacon strips to a cutting board and let it rest.

7. Add seasoned cabbage wedges into the fryer basket, close with its lid, then cook for 8 minutes at 400°F, flip the cabbage, spray with oil and continue air frying for 6 minutes until nicely golden and cooked.

8. When done, transfer cabbage wedges to a plate.

9. Chop the bacon, sprinkle it over cabbage and serve.

Nutrition:

- Calories: 123

- Carbs: 2 g

- Fat: 11 g

- Protein: 4 g

- Fiber: 0 g

- Sugar: 1g

Buffalo Cauliflower Wings

Preparation Time: 5 minutes

Cooking Time: 30 minutes

Servings: 6

Ingredients:

- 1 tablespoon of almond flour

- 1 medium head of cauliflower

- 1 ½ teaspoon of salt

- 4 tablespoons of hot sauce

- 1 tablespoon of olive oil

Directions:

1. Switch on the Air Fryer, insert fryer basket, grease it with olive oil, then shut with its lid, set the fryer to 400°F, and preheat for 5 minutes.

2. Meanwhile, cut cauliflower into bite-size florets and set aside.

3. Place flour in a large bowl, whisk in salt, oil, and hot sauce until combined, add cauliflower florets and toss until combined.

4. Open the fryer, add cauliflower florets in it in a single layer, close with its lid and cook for 15 minutes until nicely golden and crispy, shaking halfway through the frying.

5. When the Air Fryer beeps, open its lid, transfer cauliflower florets onto a serving plate and keep warm.

6. Cook the remaining cauliflower florets the same way and serve.

Nutrition:

- Calories: 48

- Carbs: 1 g

- Fat: 4 g

- Protein: 1 g

- Fiber: 0.5 g

Sweet Potato Cauliflower Patties

Preparation Time: 20 minutes

Cooking Time: 40 minutes

Servings: 7

Ingredients:

- 1 green onion, chopped

- 1 large sweet potato, peeled

- 1 teaspoon of minced garlic

- 1 cup of cilantro leaves

- 2 cup of cauliflower florets

- ¼ teaspoon of ground black pepper

- 1/4 teaspoon of salt

- 1/4 cup of sunflower seeds

- 1/4 teaspoon of cumin

- 1/4 cup of ground flaxseed

- 1/2 teaspoon of red chili powder

- 2 tablespoons of ranch seasoning mix

- 2 tablespoons of arrowroot starch

Directions:

1. Cut peeled sweet potato into small pieces, then place them in a food processor and pulse until pieces are broken up.

2. Then add onion, cauliflower florets, and garlic, pulse until combined, add remaining ingredients and pulse more until well combined.

3. Tip the mixture in a bowl, shape the mixture into seven 1 ½ inch thick patties, each about ¼ cup, then place them on a baking sheet and freeze for 10 minutes.

4. Switch on the Air Fryer, insert fryer basket, grease it with olive oil, then shut with its lid, set the fryer at 400°F, and preheat for 10 minutes.

5. Open the fryer, add patties to it in a single layer, close with its lid and cook for 20 minutes until nicely golden and cooked, flipping the patties halfway through the frying.

6. When the Air Fryer beeps, open its lid, transfer patties onto a serving plate, and keep them warm.

7. Prepare the continuing patties the same way and serve.

Nutrition:

- Calories: 85

- Carbs: 9 g

- Fat: 3 g

- Protein: 2.7 g

- Fiber: 3.5 g

Okra

Preparation Time: 10 minutes

Cooking Time: 10 minutes

Servings: 4

Ingredients:

- 1 cup of almond flour

- 8 ounces of fresh okra

- 1/2 teaspoon of sea salt

- 1 cup of milk, reduced-fat

- 1 egg, pastured

Directions:

1. Snap the egg in a basin, pour in the milk, and whisk until blended.

2. Cut the stem from each okra, then cut it into ½-inch pieces, add them into the egg and stir until well coated.

3. Mix flour and salt and add it into a large plastic bag.

4. Working on one okra piece at a time, drain the okra well by letting excess egg drip off, add it to the flour mixture, then seal the bag and shake well until okra is well coated.

5. Place the coated okra on a grease Air Fryer basket, coat the remaining okra pieces the same way and place them into the basket.

6. Switch on the Air Fryer, insert fryer basket, spray okra with oil, then shut with its lid, set the fryer to 390°F, and cook for 10 minutes until nicely golden and cooked, stirring okra halfway through the frying.

7. Serve straight away.

Nutrition:

- Calories: 250

- Carbs: 38 g

- Fat: 9 g

- Protein: 3 g

- Fiber: 2 g

Creamed Spinach

Preparation Time: 10 minutes

Cooking Time: 20 minutes

Servings: 2

Ingredients:

- 1/2 cup of chopped white onion

- 10 ounces of frozen spinach, thawed

- 1 teaspoon of salt

- 1 teaspoon of ground black pepper

- 2 teaspoons of minced garlic

- 1/2 teaspoon of ground nutmeg

- 4 ounces of cream cheese, reduced-fat, diced

- 1/4 cup of shredded Parmesan cheese, reduced-fat

Directions:

1. Switch on the Air Fryer, insert fryer basket, grease it with olive oil, then shut with its lid, set the fryer at 350°F, and preheat for 5 minutes.

2. Meanwhile, take a 6-inches baking pan, grease it with oil, and set it aside.

3. Put spinach in a basin, add remaining ingredients except for Parmesan cheese, stir until well mixed and then add the mixture into a prepared baking pan.

4. Open the fryer, add pan in it, close with its lid and cook for 10 minutes until cooked and cheese has melted, stirring halfway through.

5. Then sprinkle Parmesan cheese on top of spinach and continue air frying for 5 minutes at 400°F until the top is nicely golden and cheese has melted.

6. Serve straight away.

Nutrition:

- Calories: 273

- Carbs: 8 g

- Fat: 23 g

- Protein: 8 g

- Fiber: 2 g

Eggplant Parmesan

Preparation Time: 20 minutes

Cooking Time: 15 minutes

Servings: 4

Ingredients:

- 1/2 cup and 3 tablespoons almond flour, divided

- 1.25-pound eggplant, ½-inch sliced

- 1 tablespoon of chopped parsley

- 1 teaspoon of Italian seasoning

- 2 teaspoons of salt

- 1 cup of marinara sauce

- 1 egg, pastured

- 1 tablespoon of water

- 3 tablespoons of grated Parmesan cheese, reduced-fat

- 1/4 cup of grated mozzarella cheese, reduced-fat

Directions:

1. Slice the eggplant into ½-inch pieces, place them in a colander, sprinkle with 1 ½ teaspoon salt on both sides, and let it rest for 15 minutes.

2. Meanwhile, place ½ cup flour in a bowl, add egg and water and whisk until blended.

3. Place remaining flour in a shallow dish, add remaining salt, Italian seasoning, and Parmesan cheese, and stir until mixed.

4. Switch on the Air Fryer, insert fryer basket, grease it with olive oil, then shut with its lid, set the fryer to 360°F, and preheat for 5 minutes.

5. Meanwhile, drain the eggplant pieces, pat them dry, and then dip each slice into the egg mixture and coat with flour mixture.

6. Open the Air fryer, add coated eggplant slices in it in a single layer, close with its lid and cook for 8 minutes until nicely golden and cooked, flipping the eggplant slices halfway through the frying.

7. Then top each eggplant slice with a tablespoon of marinara sauce and some of the Mozzarella cheese and continue air frying for 1 to 2 minutes or until cheese has melted.

8. When the Air Fryer beeps, open its lid, transfer eggplants onto a serving plate, and keep them warm.

9. Cook the remaining eggplant slices the same way and serve.

Nutrition:

- Calories: 193

- Carbs: 27 g

- Fat: 5.5 g

- Protein: 10 g

- Fiber: 6 g

Cauliflower Rice

Preparation Time: 10 minutes

Cooking Time: 27 minutes

Servings: 3

Ingredients:

For the Tofu:

- 1 cup of diced carrot

- 6 ounces of tofu, extra-firm, drained

- 1/2 cup of diced white onion

- 2 tablespoons of soy sauce

- 1 teaspoon of turmeric

For the Cauliflower:

- 1/2 cup of chopped broccoli

- 3 cups of cauliflower rice

- 1 tablespoon of minced garlic

- 1/2 cup of frozen peas

- 1 tablespoon of minced ginger

- 2 tablespoons of soy sauce

- 1 tablespoon of apple cider vinegar

- 1 1/2 teaspoons of toasted sesame oil

Directions:

1. Switch on the Air Fryer, insert fryer pan, grease it with olive oil, then shut with its lid, set the fryer to 370°F, and preheat for 5 minutes.

2. Meanwhile, place tofu in a bowl, crumble it, then add remaining ingredients and stir until mixed.

3. Open the fryer, add tofu mixture in it, and spray with oil; close with its lid and cook for 10 minutes until nicely golden and crispy, stirring halfway through the frying.

4. Meanwhile, place all the ingredients for cauliflower in a bowl and toss until mixed.

5. When the Air Fryer beeps, open its lid, add cauliflower mixture, shake the pan gently to mix, and continue cooking for 12 minutes, shaking halfway through the frying.

6. Serve straight away.

Nutrition:

- Calories: 258.1

- Carbs: 20.8 g

- Fat: 13 g

- Protein: 18.2 g

- Fiber: 7 g

Brussels Sprouts

Preparation Time: 5 minutes

Cooking Time: 10 minutes

Servings: 2

Ingredients:

- 2 cups of Brussels sprouts

- 1/4 teaspoon of sea salt

- 1 tablespoon of olive oil

- 1 tablespoon of apple cider vinegar

Directions:

1. Switch on the Air Fryer, insert fryer basket, grease it with olive oil, then shut with its lid, set the fryer to 400 °F, and preheat for 5 minutes.

2. Meanwhile, cut the sprouts lengthwise into ¼-inch thick pieces, put them in a bowl, add remaining ingredients and toss until well coated.

3. Open the fryer, add sprouts in it, close with its lid and cook for 10 minutes until crispy and cooked, shaking halfway through the frying.

4. When Air Fryer beeps, open its lid, transfer sprouts onto a serving plate and serve.

Nutrition:

- Calories: 88

- Carbs: 11 g

- Fat: 4.4 g

- Protein: 3.9 g

- Fiber: 4 g

Green Beans

Preparation Time: 5 minutes

Cooking Time: 13 minutes

Servings: 4

Ingredients:

- 1-pound of green beans

- ¾ teaspoon of garlic powder

- ¾ teaspoon of ground black pepper

- 1 ¼ teaspoon of salt

- ½ teaspoon of paprika

Directions:

1. Switch on the Air Fryer, insert fryer basket, grease it with olive oil, then shut with its lid, set the fryer to 400°F, and preheat for 5 minutes.

2. Meanwhile, place the beans in a bowl, spray generously with olive oil, sprinkle with garlic powder, black pepper, salt, and paprika and toss until well coated.

3. Open the fryer, add green beans in it, close with its lid and cook for 8 minutes until nicely golden and crispy, shaking halfway through the frying.

4. When Air Fryer beeps, open its lid, transfer green beans onto a serving plate and serve.

Nutrition:

- Calories: 45

- Carbs: 7 g

- Fat: 1 g

- Protein: 2 g

- Fiber: 3 g

Asparagus Avocado Soup

Preparation Time: 10 minutes

Cooking Time: 20 minutes

Servings: 4

Ingredients:

- 1 avocado, peeled, pitted, cubed

- 12 ounces of asparagus

- ½ teaspoon of ground black pepper

- 1 teaspoon of garlic powder

- 1 teaspoon of sea salt

- 2 tablespoons of olive oil, divided

- 1/2 of a lemon, juiced

- 2 cups of vegetable stock

Directions:

1. Switch on the Air Fryer, insert fryer basket, grease it with olive oil, then shut with its lid, set the fryer to 425°F, and preheat for 5 minutes.

2. Meanwhile, place asparagus in a shallow dish, drizzle with 1 tablespoon oil, sprinkle with garlic powder, salt, and black pepper and toss until well mixed.

3. Open the fryer, add asparagus in it, close with its lid and cook for 10 minutes until nicely golden and roasted, shaking halfway through the frying.

4. When Air Fryer beeps, open its lid and transfer asparagus to a food processor.

5. Add remaining ingredients into a food processor and pulse until well combined and smooth.

6. Tip the soup in a saucepan, pour in water if the soup is too thick and heat it over medium-low heat for 5 minutes until thoroughly heated.

7. Ladle soup into bowls and serve.

Nutrition:

- Calories: 208

- Carbs: 13 g

- Fat: 16 g

- Protein: 6 g

- Fiber: 5 g

Fried Peppers with Sriracha Mayo

Preparation Time: 20 minutes

Cooking Time: 10 minutes

Servings: 2

Ingredients:

- 4 bell peppers, seeded and sliced (1-inch pieces

- 1 onion, sliced (1-inch pieces

- 1 tablespoon of olive oil

- 1/2 teaspoon of dried rosemary

- 1/2 teaspoon of dried basil

- Kosher salt, to taste

- 1/4 teaspoon of ground black pepper

- 1/3 cup of mayonnaise

- 1/3 teaspoon of Sriracha

Directions:

1. Toss the bell peppers and orions with the olive oil, rosemary, basil, salt, and black pepper.

2. Place the peppers and onions on an even layer in the cooking basket. Cook at 400°F for 12 to 14 minutes.

3. Meanwhile, make the sauce by whisking the mayonnaise and Sriracha. Serve immediately.

Nutrition:

- Calories: 346

- Fat: 34.1g

- Carbs: 9.5g

- Protein: 2.3g

- Sugars: 4.9g

Classic Fried Pickles

Preparation Time: 20 minutes

Cooking Time: 10 minutes

Servings: 2

Ingredients:

- 1 egg, whisked

- 2 tablespoons of buttermilk

- 1/2 cup of fresh breadcrumbs

- 1/4 cup of Romano cheese, grated

- 1/2 teaspoon of onion powder

- 1/2 teaspoon of garlic powder

- 1 ½ cups of dill pickle chips, pressed dry with kitchen towels

Mayo Sauce:

- 1/4 cup of mayonnaise

- 1/2 tablespoon of mustard

- 1/2 teaspoon of molasses

- 1 tablespoon of ketchup

- 1/4 teaspoon of ground black pepper

Directions:

1. In a shallow bowl, whisk the egg with buttermilk.

2. In another bowl, mix the breadcrumbs, cheese, onion powder, and garlic powder.

3. Dip the pickle chips in the egg mixture, then, dredge with the breadcrumb/cheese mixture.

4. Cook in the preheated Air Fryer at 400°F for 5 minutes; shake the basket and cook for 5 minutes more.

5. Meanwhile, mix all the sauce ingredients until well combined. Serve the fried pickles with the mayo sauce for dipping.

Nutrition:

- Calories: 342

- Fat: 28.5g

- Carbs: 12.5g

- Protein: 9.1g

- Sugars: 4.9g

Fried Green Beans with Pecorino Romano

Preparation Time: 15 minutes

Cooking Time: 10 minutes

Servings: 3

Ingredients:

- 2 tablespoons of buttermilk

- 1 egg

- 4 tablespoons of cornmeal

- 4 tablespoons of tortilla chips, crushed

- 4 tablespoons of Pecorino Romano cheese, finely grated

- Coarse salt and crushed black pepper, to taste

- 1 teaspoon of smoked paprika

- 12 ounces of green beans, trimmed

Directions:

1. In a shallow bowl, whisk together the buttermilk and egg.

2. In a separate bowl, combine the cornmeal, tortilla chips, Pecorino Romano cheese, salt, black pepper, and paprika.

3. Dip the green beans in the egg mixture, then, in the cornmeal/cheese mixture. Place the green beans in the lightly greased cooking basket.

4. Cook in the preheated Air Fryer at 390°F for 4 minutes. Shake the basket and cook for a further 3 minutes.

5. Taste, adjust the seasonings and serve with the dipping sauce if desired. Bon appétit!

Nutrition:

- Calories: 340

- Fat: 9.7g

- Carbs: 50.9g

- Protein: 12.8g

- Sugars: 4.7g

Spicy Roasted Potatoes

Preparation Time: 15 minutes

Cooking Time: 10 minutes

Servings: 2

Ingredients:

- 4 potatoes, peeled and cut into wedges

- 2 tablespoons of olive oil

- Salt and black pepper to taste

- 1 teaspoon of cayenne pepper

- 1/2 teaspoon of ancho chili powder

Directions:

1. Toss all the ingredients in a mixing bowl until the potatoes are well covered.

2. Transfer them to the Air Fryer basket and cook at 400°F for 6 minutes; shake the basket and cook for a further 6 minutes.

3. Serve wholehearted with your favorite sauce for dipping. Bon appétit!

Nutrition:

- Calories: 299

- Fat: 13.6g

- Carbs: 40.9g

- Protein: 4.8g

- Sugars: 1.4g

Spicy Glazed Carrots

Preparation Time: 20 minutes

Cooking Time: 10 minutes

Servings: 3

Ingredients:

- 1 pound carrots, cut into matchsticks

- 2 tablespoons of peanut oil

- 1 tablespoon of agave syrup

- 1 jalapeño, seeded and minced

- 1/4 teaspoon of dill

- 1/2 teaspoon of basil

- Salt and white pepper to taste

Directions:

1. Start by warming your Air Fryer to 380°F.

2. Toss all ingredients together and place them in the Air Fryer basket.

3. Cook for 15 minutes, shaking the basket halfway through the cooking time. Transfer to a serving platter and enjoy!

Nutrition:

- Calories: 162

- Fat: 9.3g

- Carbs: 20.1g

- Protein: 1.4g

- Sugars: 12.8g

Easy Sweet Potato Bake

Preparation Time: 35 minutes

Cooking Time: 30 minutes

Servings: 3

Ingredients:

- 1 stick butter, melted

- 1 pound of sweet potatoes, mashed

- 2 tablespoons of honey

- 2 eggs, beaten

- 1/3 cup of coconut milk

- 1/4 cup of flour

- 1/2 cup of fresh breadcrumbs

Directions:

1. Start by warming your Air Fryer to 325°F.

2. Grease a casserole dish with cooking oil.

3. In a mixing bowl, combine all ingredients, except for the breadcrumbs and 1 tablespoon of butter. Spoon the mixture into the prepared casserole dish.

4. Top with the breadcrumbs and brush the top with the remaining 1 tablespoon of butter. Bake in the preheated Air Fryer for 30 minutes. Bon appétit!

Nutrition:

- Calories: 409

- Fat: 26.1g

- Carbs: 38.3g

- Protein: 7.2g

- Sugars: 10.9g

Avocado Fries with Roasted Garlic Mayonnaise

Preparation Time: 50 minutes

Cooking Time: 1 hour

Servings: 4

Ingredients:

- 1/2 head garlic 6-7 cloves

- 3/4 cup of all-purpose flour

- Salt and black pepper to taste

- 2 eggs

- 1 cup of tortilla chips, crushed

- 3 avocados, cut into wedges

Sauce:

- 1/2 cup of mayonnaise

- 1 teaspoon of lemon juice

- 1 teaspoon of mustard

Directions:

1. Put the garlic on a piece of aluminum foil and drizzle with cooking spray. Wrap the garlic in the foil.

2. Cook in the preheated Air Fryer at 400 °F for 12 minutes. Check the garlic, open the top of the foil and continue to cook for 10 minutes more.

3. Let it rest for 10 to 15 minutes; remove the cloves by squeezing them out of the skins; mash the garlic and reserve.

4. In a shallow bowl, combine the flour, salt, and black pepper. In another shallow dish, whisk the eggs until frothy.

5. Place the crushed tortilla chips in a third shallow dish. Dredge the avocado wedges in the flour mixture, shaking off the excess. Then, dip in the egg mixture; last, dredge in crushed tortilla chips.

6. Sprinkle the avocado wedges with cooking oil on all sides.

7. Cook in the preheated Air Fryer at 395°F approximately 8 minutes, turning them over halfway through the cooking time.

8. Meanwhile, combine the sauce ingredients with the smashed roasted garlic. To serve, divide the avocado fries between plates and top with the sauce. Enjoy!

Nutrition:

- Calories: 351

- Fat: 27.7g

- Carbs: 21.5g

- Protein: 6.4g

- Sugars: 1.1g

Roasted Broccoli with Sesame Seeds

Preparation Time: 15 minutes

Cooking Time: 10 minutes

Servings: 2

Ingredients:

- 1 pound broccoli florets

- 2 tablespoons of sesame oil

- 1/2 teaspoon of shallot powder

- 1/2 teaspoon of porcini powder

- 1 teaspoon of garlic powder

- Salt and pepper to taste

- 1/2 teaspoon of cumin powder

- 1/4 teaspoon of paprika

- 2 tablespoons of sesame seeds

Directions:

1. Start by warming the Air Fryer to 400°F.

2. Blanch the broccoli in salted boiling water until al dente, about 3 to 4 minutes. Drain well and transfer to the lightly greased Air Fryer basket.

3. Add the sesame oil, shallot powder, porcini powder, garlic powder, salt, black pepper, cumin powder, paprika, and sesame seeds.

4. Cook for 6 minutes, tossing them over halfway through the cooking time. Bon appétit!

Nutrition:

- Calories: 267

- Fat: 19.5g

- Carbs: 20.2g

- Protein: 8.9g

- Sugars: 5.2g

Corn on the Cob with Herb Butter

Preparation Time: 15 minutes

Cooking Time: 10 minutes

Servings: 2

Ingredients:

- 2 ears fresh corn, shucked and cut into halves

- 2 tablespoons of butter, room temperature

- 1 teaspoon of granulated garlic

- 1/2 teaspoon of fresh ginger, grated

- Salt and pepper to taste

- 1 tablespoon of fresh rosemary, chopped

- 1 tablespoon of fresh basil, chopped

- 2 tablespoons of fresh chives, roughly chopped

Directions:

1. Spray the corn with cooking spray. Cook at 395ºF for 6 minutes, turning them over halfway through the cooking time.

2. In the meantime, mix the butter with the granulated: garlic, ginger, salt, black pepper, rosemary, and basil.

3. Spread the butter mixture all over the corn on the cob. Cook in the preheated Air Fryer an additional 2 minutes. Bon appétit!

Nutrition:

- Calories: 239

- Fat: 13.3g

- Carbs: 30.2g

- Protein: 5.4g

- Sugars: 5.8g

Rainbow Vegetable Fritters

Preparation Time: 20 minutes

Cooking Time: 10 minutes

Servings: 2

Ingredients:

- 1 zucchini, grated and squeezed

- 1 cup of corn kernels

- 1/2 cup of canned green peas

- 4 tablespoons of all-purpose flour

- 2 tablespoons of fresh shallots, minced

- 1 teaspoon of fresh garlic, minced

- 1 tablespoon of peanut oil

- Salt and pepper to taste

- 1 teaspoon of cayenne pepper

Directions:

1. In a mixing bowl, thoroughly combine all the ingredients until everything is well combined.

2. Shape the mixture into patties. Spray the Air Fryer basket with cooking spray.

3. Cook in the preheated Air Fryer at 365°F for 6 minutes. Turn them over and cook for a further 6 minutes.

4. Serve immediately and enjoy!

Nutrition:

- Calories: 215

- Fat: 8.4g

- Carbs: 31.6g

- Protein: 6g

- Sugars: 4.1g

Cauliflower and Goat Cheese Croquettes

Preparation Time: 30 minutes

Cooking Time: 26 minutes

Servings: 2

Ingredients:

- 1/2 pound of cauliflower florets

- 2 garlic cloves, minced

- 1 cup of goat cheese, shredded

- Salt and pepper to taste

- 1/2 teaspoon of shallot powder

- 1/4 teaspoon of cumin powder

- 1 cup of sour cream

- 1 teaspoon of Dijon mustard

Directions:

1. Put the cauliflower florets in a saucepan of water; bring to the boil; reduce the heat and cook for 10 minutes or until tender.

2. Mash the cauliflower using your blender; add the garlic, cheese, and spices; mix to combine well.

3. Form the cauliflower mixture into croquettes shapes.

4. Cook in the preheated Air Fryer at 375°F for 16 minutes, shaking halfway through the cooking time. Serve with the sour cream and mustard. Bon appétit!

Nutrition:

- Calories: 297

- Fat: 21.7g

- Carbs: 11.7g

- Protein: 15.3g

- Sugars: 2.6g

Chapter 5. Desserts and Breakfast

Pancakes

Preparation Time: 5 minutes

Cooking Time: 29 minutes

Servings: 4

Ingredients:

- 1 1/2 cup of coconut flour

- 1 teaspoon of salt

- 3 1/2 teaspoons of baking powder

- 1 tablespoon of Erythritol sweetener

- 1 1/2 teaspoon of baking soda

- 3 tablespoons of melted butter

- 1 1/4 cups of milk, unsweetened, reduced-fat

- 1 egg, pastured

Directions:

1. Switch on the Air Fryer, insert fryer pan, grease it with olive oil, then shut with its lid, set the fryer to 220°F, and preheat for 5 minutes.

2. Meanwhile, take a medium bowl, add all the ingredients in it, whisk until well blended and then let the mixture rest for 5 minutes.

3. Open the fryer, pour in some of the pancake mixture as thin as possible, close with its lid and cook for 6 minutes until nicely golden, turning the pancake halfway through the frying.

4. When Air Fryer beeps, open its lid, transfer pancake onto a serving plate and use the remaining batter for cooking more pancakes the same way.

5. Serve straight away with fresh fruits slices.

Nutrition:

- Calories: 237.7 Cal

- Carbs: 39.2 g

- Fat: 10.2 g

- Protein: 6.3 g

- Fiber: 1.3 g

Zucchini Bread

Preparation Time: 25 minutes

Cooking Time: 40 minutes

Servings: 8

Ingredients:

- ¾ cup of shredded zucchini

- 1/2 cup of almond flour

- 1/4 teaspoon of salt

- 1/4 cup of cocoa powder, unsweetened

- 1/2 cup of chocolate chips, unsweetened, divided

- 6 tablespoons of Erythritol sweetener

- 1/2 teaspoon of baking soda

- 2 tablespoons of olive oil

- 1/2 teaspoon of vanilla extract, unsweetened

- 2 tablespoons of butter, unsalted, melted

- 1 egg, pastured

Directions:

1. Switch on the Air Fryer, insert fryer basket, grease it with olive oil, then shut with its lid, set the fryer to 310°F, and preheat for 10 minutes.

2. Meanwhile, place flour in a bowl, add salt, cocoa powder, and baking soda and stir until mixed.

3. Crack the eggs in another bowl, whisk in sweetener, egg, oil, butter, and vanilla until smooth and then slowly whisk in flour mixture until well combined.

4. Add zucchini along with 1/3 cup chocolate chips and then fold until just mixed.

5. Take a mini loaf pan that fits into the Air Fryer, grease it with olive oil, then pour in the prepared batter and sprinkle remaining chocolate chips on top.

6. Open the fryer, place the loaf pan in it, close with its lid and cock for 30 minutes at the 310 °F until inserted toothpick into the bread slides comes out clean.

7. When Air Fryer beeps, open its lid, remove the loaf pan, then place it on a wire rack and let the bread cool in it for 20 minutes.

8. Take out the bread, let it cool completely, then cut it into slices and serve.

Nutrition:

- Calories: 356 Cal

- Carbs: 49 g

- Fat: 17 g

- Protein: 5.1 g

- Fiber: 2.5 g

Blueberry Muffins

Preparation Time: 10 minutes

Cooking Time: 30 minutes

Servings: 14

Ingredients:

- 1 cup of almond flour

- 1 cup of frozen blueberries

- 2 teaspoons of baking powder

- 1/3 cup of Erythritol sweetener

- 1 teaspoon of vanilla extract, unsweetened

- ½ teaspoon of salt

- ¼ cup of melted coconut oil

- 1 egg, pastured

- ¼ cup of applesauce, unsweetened

- ¼ cup of almond milk, unsweetened

Directions:

1. Switch on the Air Fryer, insert fryer basket, grease it with olive oil, then shut with its lid, set the fryer at 360°F, and preheat for 10 minutes.

2. Meanwhile, place flour in a large bowl, add blueberries, salt, sweetener, baking powder, and stir until well combined.

3. Crack the eggs in another bowl, whisk in vanilla, milk, and applesauce until combined, and then slowly whisk in flour mixture until well combined.

4. Take fourteen silicone muffin cups, grease them with oil, and then evenly fill them with the prepared batter.

5. Open the fryer; stack muffin cups in it, close with its lid, and cook for 10 minutes until muffins are nicely golden brown and set.

6. When the Air Fryer beeps, open its lid, transfer muffins onto a serving plate, and then remaining muffins in the same manner.

7. Serve straight away.

Nutrition:

- Calories: 201 Cal

- Carbs: 27.3 g

- Fat: 8.8 g

- Protein: 3 g

- Fiber: 1.2 g

Baked Eggs

Preparation Time: 5 minutes

Cooking Time: 17 minutes

Servings: 2

Ingredients:

- 2 tablespoons of frozen spinach, thawed

- ½ teaspoon of salt

- ¼ teaspoon of ground black pepper

- 2 eggs, pastured

- 3 teaspoons of grated Parmesan cheese, reduced-fat

- 2 tablespoons of milk, unsweetened, reduced-fat

Directions:

1. Switch on the Air Fryer, insert fryer basket, grease it with olive oil, then shut with its lid, set the fryer at 330°F, and preheat for 5 minutes.

2. Meanwhile, take two silicon muffin cups, grease them with oil, then crack an egg into each cup and evenly add cheese, spinach, and milk.

3. Season the egg with salt and black pepper and gently stir the ingredients without breaking the egg yolk.

4. Open the fryer, add muffin cups to it, close with its lid and cook for 8 to 12 minutes until eggs have cooked to desired doneness.

5. When the Air Fryer beeps, open its lid, take out the muffin cups and serve.

Nutrition:

- Calories: 161 Cal

- Carbs: 3 g

- Fat: 11.4 g

- Protein: 12.1 g

- Fiber: 1.1 g

Bagels

Preparation Time: 10 minutes

Cooking Time: 20 minutes

Servings: 6

Ingredients:

- 2 cups of almond flour

- 2 cups of shredded mozzarella cheese, low-fat

- 2 tablespoons of butter, unsalted

- 1 1/2 teaspoon of baking powder

- 1 teaspoon of apple cider vinegar

- 1 egg, pastured

For Egg Wash:

- 1 egg, pastured

- 1 teaspoon butter, unsalted, melted

Directions:

1. Place flour in a heatproof bowl, add cheese and butter, then stir well and microwave for 90 seconds until butter and cheese has melted.

2. Then stir the mixture until well combined, let it cool for 5 minutes and whisk in the egg, baking powder, and vinegar until well combined and the dough comes together.

3. Let the dough cool for 10 minutes, then divide the dough into six sections, shape each section into a bagel and let the bagels rest for 5 minutes.

4. Prepare the egg wash and for this, place the melted butter in a bowl, whisk in the egg until blended, and then brush the mixture generously on top of each bagel.

5. Take a fryer basket, line it with parchment paper, and then place prepared bagels in it in a single layer.

6. Switch on the Air Fryer, insert fryer, then shut with its lid, set the fryer to 350°F, and cook for 10 minutes at 350°F until bagels are nicely golden and thoroughly cooked, turning the bagels halfway through the frying.

7. When the Air Fryer beeps, open its lid, transfer bagels to a serving plate, and cook the remaining bagels the same way.

8. Serve straight away.

Nutrition:

- Calories: 408.7 Cal

- Carbs: 8.3 g

- Fat: 33.5 g

- Protein: 20.3 g

- Fiber: 4 g

Cauliflower Hash Browns

Preparation Time: 10 minutes

Cooking Time: 25 minutes

Servings: 6

Ingredients:

- 1/4 cup of chickpea flour

- 4 cups of cauliflower rice

- 1/2 medium white onion, peeled and chopped

- 1/2 teaspoon of garlic powder

- 1 tablespoon of xanthan gum

- 1/2 teaspoon of salt

- 1 tablespoon of nutritional yeast flakes

- 1 teaspoon of ground paprika

Directions:

1. Switch on the Air Fryer, insert fryer basket, grease it with olive oil, then shut with its lid, set the fryer to 375°F, and preheat for 10 minutes.

2. Meanwhile, place all the ingredients in a bowl, stir until well mixed and then shape the mixture into six rectangular disks, each about ½-inch thick.

3. Open the fryer, add hash browns in it in a single layer, close with its lid and cook for 25 minutes at 375°F until nicely golden and crispy, turning halfway through the frying.

4. When the Air Fryer beeps, open its lid, transfer hash browns to a serving plate and serve.

Nutrition:

- Calories: 115.2 Cal

- Carbs: 6.2 g

- Fat: 7.3 g

- Protein: 7.4 g

- Fiber: 2.2 g

Chicken Sandwich

Preparation Time: 40 minutes

Cooking Time: 20 minutes

Servings: 6

Ingredients:

- 4 chicken breasts, pastured

- 1 cup of almond flour

- ¾ teaspoon of ground black pepper

- 1/2 teaspoon of paprika

- 1 teaspoon of salt

- 1/2 teaspoon of celery seeds

- 1 teaspoon of potato starch

- 1/4 cup of milk, reduced-fat

- 4 cups of dill pickle juice as needed

- 2 eggs, pastured

- 4 hamburger buns

- 1/8 teaspoon of dry milk powder, nonfat

- ¼ teaspoon of xanthan gum

- 1/8 teaspoon of Erythritol sweetener

Directions:

1. Place the chicken in a large plastic bag, seal the bag and then pound the chicken with a mallet until ½-inch thick.

2. Brine the chicken and for this, pour the dill, pickle juice in the plastic bag containing chicken, then seal it and let the chicken soak for a minimum of 2 hours.

3. After 2 hours, remove the chicken from the brine, rinse it well, and pat dry with paper towels.

4. Place flour in a shallow dish, add black pepper, paprika, salt, celery, potato starch, milk powder, xanthan gum, sweetener, and stir until well mixed.

5. Crack eggs in another dish and then whisk until blended.

6. Switch on the Air Fryer, insert fryer basket, grease it with olive oil, then shut with its lid, set the fryer to 375°F, and preheat for 5 minutes.

7. Meanwhile, dip the chicken into the egg and then coat evenly with the flour mixture.

8. Open the fryer, add chicken breasts to it in a single layer, close with its lid, then cook for 10 minutes, flip the chickens and continue cooking for 5 minutes or until chicken is nicely golden and cooked.

9. When the Air Fryer beeps, open its lid, transfer chicken to a plate, and cook the remaining chicken the same way.

10. Sandwich a chicken breast between toasted hamburger buns, top with favorite dressing, and serve.

Nutrition:

- Calories: 440 Cal

- Carbs: 40 g

- Fat: 19 g

- Protein: 28 g

- Fiber: 12 g

Tofu Scramble

Preparation Time: 5 minutes

Cooking Time: 18 minutes

Servings: 3

Ingredients:

- 12 ounces of tofu, extra-firm, drained, ½-inch cubed

- 1 teaspoon of garlic powder

- 1 teaspoon of onion powder

- 1 teaspoon of paprika

- 1/2 teaspoon of ground black pepper

- 1/2 teaspoon of salt

- 1 tablespoon of olive oil

- 2 teaspoon of xanthan gum

Directions:

1. Switch on the Air Fryer, insert fryer basket, grease it with olive oil, then shut with its lid, set the fryer at 220°F, and preheat for 5 minutes.

2. Meanwhile, place tofu pieces in a bowl, drizzle with oil, and sprinkle with xanthan gum and toss until well coated.

3. Add remaining ingredients to the tofu and then toss until well coated.

4. Open the fryer, add tofu to it, close with its lid and cook for 13 minutes until nicely golden and crispy, shaking the basket every 5 minutes.

5. When the Air Fryer beeps, open its lid, transfer tofu onto a serving plate and serve.

Nutrition:

- Calories: 94 Cal

- Carbs: 5 g

- Fat: 5 g

- Protein: 6 g

- Fiber: 0 g

Fried Egg

Preparation Time: 5 minutes

Cooking Time: 4 minutes

Servings: 1

Ingredients:

- 1 egg, pastured

- 1/8 teaspoon of salt

- 1/8 teaspoon of cracked black pepper

Directions:

1. Take the fryer pan, grease it with olive oil and then crack the egg in it.

2. Switch on the Air Fryer, insert fryer pan, then shut with its lid, and set the fryer to 370°F.

3. Set the frying time to 3 minutes, then when the Air Fryer beep, open its lid and check the egg; if the egg needs more cooking, then Air Fryer it for another minute.

4. Transfer the egg to a serving plate, season with salt and black pepper, and serve.

Nutrition:

- Calories: 90 Cal

- Carbs: 0.6 g

- Fat: 7 g

- Protein: 6.3 g

- Fiber: 0 g

Cheesecake Bites

Preparation Time: 40 minutes

Cooking Time: 9 minutes

Servings: 4

Ingredients:

- 1/2 cup of almond flour

- 1/2 cup of and 2 tablespoons Erythritol sweetener, divided

- 8 ounces of cream cheese, reduced-fat, softened

- 1/2 teaspoon of vanilla extract, unsweetened

- 4 tablespoons of heavy cream, reduced-fat, divided

Directions:

1. Prepare the cheesecake mixture, and for this, place softened cream cheese in a bowl, add cream, vanilla, and ½-cup of sweetener and whisk using an electric mixer until smooth.

2. Scoop the mixture on a baking sheet lined with parchment sheet, then place it in the freezer for 30 minutes until firm.

3. Place flour in a small bowl and stir in the remaining sweetener.

4. Then switch on the Air Fryer, insert fryer basket, grease it with olive oil, then shut with its lid, set the fryer at 350°F, and preheat for 5 minutes.

5. Meanwhile, cut the cheesecake mix into bite-size pieces and then coat it with an almond flour mixture.

6. Open the fryer, add cheesecake bites in it, close with its lid and cook for 2 minutes until nicely golden and crispy.

7. Serve straight away.

Nutrition:

- Calories: 198 Cal

- Carbs: 6 g

- Fat: 18 g

- Protein: 3 g

- Fiber: 0 g

Coconut Pie

Preparation Time: 5 minutes

Cooking Time: 45 minutes

Servings: 6

Ingredients:

- 1/2 cup of coconut flour

- 1/2 cup of Erythritol sweetener

- 1 cup of shredded coconut, unsweetened, divided

- 1/4 cup of butter, unsalted

- 1 1/2 teaspoon of vanilla extract, unsweetened

- 2 eggs, pastured

- 1 1/2 cups of milk, low-fat, unsweetened

- ¼ cup of shredded coconut, toasted

Directions:

1. Switch on the Air Fryer, insert fryer basket, grease it with olive oil, then shut with its lid, set the fryer to 350°F, and preheat for 5 minutes.

2. Meanwhile, place all the ingredients in a bowl and whisk until well blended and smooth batter comes together.

3. Take a 6-inches pie pan, grease it oil, then pour in the prepared batter and smooth the top.

4. Open the fryer, place the pie pan in it, close with its lid, and cook for 45 minutes until pie has set and when inserted a toothpick into the pie, it slides out clean.

5. When the Air Fryer beeps, open its lid, take out the pie pan and let it cool.

6. Garnish the pie with toasted coconut, then cut into slices and serve.

Nutrition:

- Calories: 236 Cal

- Carbs: 16 g

- Fat: 16 g

- Protein: 3 g

- Fiber: 2 g

Crust less Cheesecake

Preparation Time: 5 minutes

Cooking Time: 10 minutes

Servings: 2

Ingredients:

- 16 ounces of cream cheese, reduced-fat, softened

- 2 tablespoons of sour cream, reduced-fat

- 3/4 cup of Erythritol sweetener

- 1 teaspoon of vanilla extract, unsweetened

- 2 eggs, pastured

- 1/2 teaspoon of lemon juice

Directions:

1. Switch on the Air Fryer, insert fryer basket, grease it with olive oil, then shut with its lid, set the fryer to 350°F, and preheat for 5 minutes.

2. Meanwhile, take two 4 inches of spring form pans, grease them with oil, and set them aside.

3. Crack the eggs in a bowl and then whisk in lemon juice, sweetener and vanilla until smooth.

4. Whisk in cream cheese and sour cream until blended, and then divide the mixture evenly between prepared pans.

5. Open the fryer, place pans in it, close with its lid, and cook for 10 minutes until cakes are set and an inserted skewer into the cakes slides out clean.

6. When the Air Fryer beeps, open its lid. Please take out the cake pans and let the cakes cool in them.

7. Take out the cakes, refrigerate for 3 hours until cooled, and then serve.

Nutrition:

- Calories: 318 Cal

- Carbs: 1 g

- Fat: 29.7 g

- Protein: 11.7 g

- Fiber: 0 g

Chocolate Cake

Preparation Time: 5 minutes

Cooking Time: 15 minutes

Servings: 6

Ingredients:

- 1/4 cup of coconut flour

- 1 teaspoon of baking powder

- 1/3 cup of Truvia sweetener

- 1/4 teaspoon of salt

- 2 tablespoon of cocoa powder, unsweetened

- 1 teaspoon of vanilla extract, unsweetened

- 4 tablespoons of butter, unsalted, melted

- 3 eggs, pastured

- 1/2 cup of heavy whipping cream, reduced-fat

Directions:

1. Switch on the Air Fryer, insert fryer basket, grease it with olive oil, then shut with its lid, set the fryer to 350°F, and preheat for 5 minutes.

2. Meanwhile, take a 6 cups muffin pan, grease it with oil, and set aside until required.

3. Place melted butter in a bowl, whisk in sweetener until blended, and then beat in vanilla, eggs, and cream until combined.

4. Add remaining ingredients, beat again until well combined and smooth batter comes together, and then pour the mixture into the prepared pan.

5. Open the fryer, place the pan in it, close with its lid and cook for 10 minutes until the cake is done and an inserted skewer into the cake slides out clean.

6. When the Air Fryer beeps, open its lid, take out the cake pan and let the cake cool in it.

7. Please, take out the cakes, cut them into pieces, and serve.

Nutrition:

- Calories: 192 Cal

- Carbs: 8 g

- Fat: 16 g

- Protein: 4 g

- Fiber: 2 g

Chocolate Brownies

Preparation Time: 10 minutes

Cooking Time: 45 minutes

Servings: 4

Ingredients:

- 1/2 cup of chocolate chips, sugar-free

- 1 teaspoon of vanilla extract, unsweetened

- 1/4 cup of Erythritol sweetener

- 1/2 cup of butter, unsalted

- 3 eggs, pastured

Directions:

1. Switch on the Air Fryer, insert fryer basket, grease it with olive oil, then shut with its lid, set the fryer to 350°F, and preheat for 10 minutes.

2. Meanwhile, place chocolate and butter in a heatproof bowl and microwave for 1 minute or until chocolate has melted, stirring every 30 seconcs.

3. Crack eggs in another bowl, beat in vanilla and sweetener until smooth, and then slowly beat in melted chocolate mixture until well combined.

4. Take a spring-form pan that fist into the Air Fryer, grease it with oil, and then pour in batter in it.

5. Open the fryer, place the pan in it, close with its lid, and cook for 35 minutes until the cake is done and an inserted toothpick into the brownies slides out clean.

6. When the Air Fryer beeps, open its lid. Please take out the pan and let the brownies cool in it.

7. Then take out the brownies, cut them into even pieces, and serve.

Nutrition:

- Calories: 224 Cal

- Carbs: 3 g

- Fat: 23 g

- Protein: 4 g

- Fiber: 1 g

Spiced Apples

Preparation Time: 5 minutes

Cooking Time: 17 minutes

Servings: 4

Ingredients:

- 4 small apples, cored, sliced

- 2 tablespoons of Erythritol sweetener

- 1 teaspoon of apple pie spice

- 2 tablespoons of olive oil

Directions:

1. Switch on the Air Fryer, insert fryer basket, grease it with olive oil, then shut with its lid, set the fryer to 350°F, and preheat for 5 minutes.

2. Meanwhile, place apple slice in a bowl, sprinkle with sweetener and spice, and drizzle with oil and stir until evenly coated.

3. Open the Fryer, add apple slices in it, close with its lid and cook for 12 minutes until nicely golden and crispy, shaking halfway through the frying.

4. Serve straight away.

Nutrition:

- Calories: 89.6 Cal

- Carbs: 21.8 g

- Fat: 2 g

- Protein: 0.5 g

- Fiber: 5.3 g

Pumpkin Custard

Preparation Time: 2 hours 30 minutes

Cooking Time: 0

Servings: 6

Ingredients:

- 1/2 cup of almond flour

- 4 eggs

- 1 cup of pumpkin puree

- 1/2 cup of stevia/Erythritol blend, granulated

- 1/8 teaspoon of sea salt

- 1 teaspoon of vanilla extract or maple flavoring

- 4 tablespoons of butter, ghee, or coconut oil melted

- 1 teaspoon of pumpkin pie spice

Directions:

1. Grease or spray a slow cooker with butter or coconut oil spray.

2. In a medium mixing bowl, beat the eggs until smooth. Then add in the sweetener.

3. To the egg mixture, add in the pumpkin puree along with vanilla or maple extract.

4. Then add almond flour to the mixture along with the pumpkin pie spice and salt. Add melted butter, coconut oil, or ghee.

5. Transfer the mixture into a slow cooker. Close the lid. Cook for 2-2 ¾ hours on Low.

6. When through, serve with whipped cream, and then sprinkle with little nutmeg if needed. Enjoy!

7. Set slow-cooker to the Low setting. Cook for 2-2.45 hours, and begin checking at the two-hour mark. Serve warm with stevia-sweetened whipped cream and a sprinkle of nutmeg.

Nutrition:

- Calories: 70

- Total Fat 0.7g

- Saturated Fat 0.1g

- Total Carbs 14.7g

- Net Carbs 12.2g

- Protein 2.1g

- Sugar 2.2g

- Fiber 2.5g

- Sodium 1mg

Peanut Butter Banana "Ice Cream"

Preparation Time: 10 minutes

Cooking Time: 0

Servings: 6

Ingredients:

- 4 medium bananas

- ½ cup of whipped peanut butter

- 1-teaspoon of vanilla extract

Directions:

1. Peel the bananas and slice them into coins.

2. Arrange the slices on a plate and freeze until solid.

3. Place the frozen bananas in a food processor.

4. Add the peanut butter and mix until it is mostly smooth.

5. Scrape down the sides, then add the vanilla extract.

6. Mix until smooth, then spoon into bowls to serve.

Nutrition:

- Calories: 70

- Total Fat: 0.7g

- Saturated Fat: 0.1g

- Total Carbs: 14.7g

- Net Carbs: 12.2g

- Protein: 2.1g

- Sugar: 2.2g

- Fiber: 2.5g

- Sodium: 1mg

Fruity Coconut Energy Balls

Preparation Time: 15 minutes

Cooking Time: 0

Servings: 18

Ingredients:

- 1 cup of chopped almonds

- 1 cup of dried figs

- ½ cup of dried apricots, chopped

- ½ cup of dried cranberries, unsweetened

- ½-teaspoon of vanilla extract

- ¼-teaspoon of ground cinnamon

- ½ cup of shredded unsweetened coconut

Directions:

1. Put the almonds, figs, apricots, and cranberries in a food processor.

2. Blend the mixture until finely chopped.

3. Add the vanilla extract and cinnamon, then blend to combine once more.

4. Roll the mixture into 18 small balls by hand.

5. Roll the balls in the shredded coconut and chill until firm.

Nutrition:

- Calories: 100

- Total Fat: 0.7g

- Saturated Fat: 0.1g

- Total Carbs: 14.7g

- Net Carbs: 12.2g

- Protein: 2.1g

- Sugar: 2.2g

- Fiber 2.5g

- Sodium: 1mg

Mini Apple Oat Muffins

Preparation Time: 5minutes

Cooking Time: 25 minutes

Servings: 24

Ingredients:

- 1 ½ cups of old-fashioned oats

- 1 teaspoon of baking powder

- ½ teaspoon of ground cinnamon

- ¼ teaspoon of baking soda

- ¼ teaspoon of salt

- ½ cup of unsweetened applesauce

- ¼ cup of light brown sugar

- 3 tablespoons of canola oil

- 3 tablespoons of water

- 1 teaspoon of vanilla extract

- ½ cup of slivered almonds

Directions:

1. Preheat the oven to 350°F and grease a mini muffin pan.

2. Place the oats in a food processor and mix into a fine flour.

3. Add the baking powder, cinnamon, baking soda, and salt.

4. Mix until well combined, add the applesauce, brown sugar, canola oil, water, and vanilla and then blend smooth.

5. Fold in the almonds and spoon the mixture into the muffin pan.

6. Bake for 22 to 25 minutes until a knife inserted in the center comes out clean.

7. Cool the muffins for 5 minutes, then turn them out onto a wire rack.

Nutrition:

- Calories: 70

- Total Fat: 0.7g

- Saturated Fat: 0.1g

- Total Carbs: 14.7g

- Net Carbs: 12.2g

- Protein: 2.1g

- Sugar: 2.2g

- Fiber: 2.5g

- Sodium: 1mg

Dark Chocolate Almond Yogurt Cups

Preparation Time: 10 minutes

Cooking Time: 0

Servings: 6

Ingredients:

- 3 cups of plain nonfat Greek yogurt

- ½-teaspoon of almond extract

- ¼-teaspoon of liquid stevia extract (more to taste)

- 2 ounces 70% dark chocolate, chopped

- ½ cup of slivered almonds

Directions:

1. Whisk together the yogurt, almond extract, and liquid stevia in a medium bowl.

2. Spoon the yogurt into four dessert cups.

3. Sprinkle with chopped chocolate and slivered almonds.

Nutrition:

- Calories: 170

- Total Fat: 0.7g

- Saturated Fat: 0.1g

- Total Carbs: 14.7g

- Net Carbs: 12.2g

- Protein: 2.1g

- Sugar 2.2g

- Fiber 2.5g

- Sodium 41mg

Chocolate Avocado Mousse

Preparation Time: 5 minutes

Cooking Time: 0

Servings: 3

Ingredients:

- 1 large avocado, pitted and chopped

- ¼ cup of fat-free milk

- ¼ cup of unsweetened cocoa powder (dark)

- 2 teaspoons of powdered stevia

- 1-teaspoon of vanilla extract

- 2 tablespoons of fat-free whipped topping

Directions:

1. Place the avocado in a food processor and blend smooth.

2. In a small bowl, whisk together the milk and cocoa powder until well mixed.

3. Stir in the pureed avocado along with the stevia and vanilla extract.

4. Spoon into bowls and serve with fat-free whipped topping.

Nutrition:

- Calories 180

- Total Fat 0.7g,

- Saturated Fat 0.1g

- Total Carbs 14.7g

- Net Carbs 12.2g

- Protein 2.1g

- Sugar 2.2g

- Fiber 2.5g

- Sodium 23mg

Pumpkin Spice Snack Balls

Preparation Time: 15 minutes

Cooking Time: 10 minutes

Servings: 10

Ingredients:

- 1 ½ cups of old-fashioned oats

- ½ cup of chopped almonds

- ½ cup of unsweetened shredded coconut

- ¾ cup of canned pumpkin puree

- 2 tablespoons of honey

- 2 teaspoons of pumpkin pie spice

- ¼-teaspoon of salt

Directions:

1. Preheat the oven to 300°F and line a baking sheet with parchment.

2. Combine the oats, almonds, and coconut on the baking sheet.

3. Bake for 8 to 10 minutes until browned, stirring halfway through.

4. Place the pumpkin, honey, pumpkin pie spice, and salt in a medium bowl.

5. Stir in the toasted oat mixture.

6. Shape the mixture into 20 balls by hand and place on a tray.

7. Chill until the balls are firm, then serve.

Nutrition:

- Calories: 170

- Total Fat: 0.7g

- Saturated Fat: 0.1g

- Total Carbs: 14.7g

- Net Carbs: 12.2g

- Protein: 2.1g

- Sugar: 2.2g

- Fiber: 2.5g

- Sodium: 1mg

Strawberry Lime Pudding

Preparation Time: 15 minutes

Cooking Time: 10 minutes

Servings: 4

Ingredients:

- 2 cups plus 2 of tablespoons fat-free milk

- 2 teaspoons of flavorless gelatin

- 10 large strawberries, sliced

- 1 tablespoon of fresh lime zest

- 2 teaspoons of vanilla extract

- Liquid stevia extract, to taste

Directions:

1. Whisk together 2 tablespoons of milk and gelatin in a medium bowl until the gelatin dissolves completely.

2. Place the strawberries in a food processor with the lime juice and vanilla extract.

3. Blend until smooth, then pour into a medium bowl.

4. Warm the remaining milk in a small saucepan over medium heat.

5. Stir in the lime zest and heat until steaming (do not boil).

6. Gently whisk the gelatin mixture into the hot milk, then stir in the strawberry mixture.

7. Sweeten with liquid stevia to taste and chill until set. Serve cold.

Nutrition:

- Calories: 70

- Total Fat: 0.7g

- Saturated Fat: 0.1g

- Total Carbs: 14.7g

- Net Carbs: 12.2g

- Protein: 2.1g

- Sugar: 2.2g

- Fiber: 2.5g

- Sodium: 1mg

Cinnamon Toasted Almonds

Preparation Time: 5 minutes

Cooking Time: 25 minutes

Servings: 8

Ingredients:

- 2 cups of whole almonds

- 1-tablespoon of olive oil

- 1 teaspoon of ground cinnamon

- ½ teaspoon of salt

Directions:

1. Preheat the oven to 325°F and line a baking sheet with parchment.

2. Toss together the almonds, olive oil, cinnamon, and salt.

3. Spread the almonds on the baking sheet in a single layer.

4. Bake for 25 minutes, stirring several times until toasted.

Nutrition:

- Calories: 150

- Total Fat: 13.6g

- Saturated Fat: 1.2g

- Total Carbs: 5.3g

- Net Carbs: 2.2g

- Protein: 5g

- Sugar: 1g

- Fiber: 3.1g

- Sodium: 148mg

Grain-Free Berry Cobbler

Preparation Time: 5 minutes

Cooking Time: 25 minutes

Servings: 10

Ingredients:

- 4 cups of fresh mixed berries

- ½ cup of ground flaxseed

- ¼ cup of almond meal

- ¼ cup of unsweetened shredded coconut

- ½ tablespoon of baking powder

- 1 teaspoon of ground cinnamon

- ¼ teaspoon of salt

- Powdered stevia, to taste

- 6 tablespoons of coconut oil

Directions:

1. Preheat the oven to 375°F and lightly grease a 10-inch cast-iron skillet.

2. Spread the berries on the bottom of the skillet.

3. Whisk together the dry ingredients in a mixing bowl.

4. Cut in the coconut oil using a fork to create a crumbled mixture.

5. Spread the crumble over the berries and bake for 25 minutes until hot and bubbling.

6. Cool the cobbler for 5 to 10 minutes before serving.

Nutrition:

- Calories: 215

- Total Fat: 13.6g

- Saturated Fat: 1.2g

- Total Carbs: 5.3g

- Net Carbs: 2.2g

- Protein: 5g

- Sugar: 1g

- Fiber: 3.1g

- Sodium: 67mg

Whole-Wheat Pumpkin Muffins

Preparation Time: 15 minutes

Cooking Time: 15 minutes

Servings: 36

Ingredients:

- 1 ¾-cup of whole-wheat flour

- 1 teaspoon of baking powder

- 1 teaspoon of baking soda

- 1 teaspoon of ground cinnamon

- 1 teaspoon of pumpkin pie spice

- ½ teaspoon of salt

- 2 large eggs

- 1 cup of canned pumpkin puree

- 1/3 cup of unsweetened applesauce

- ¼ cup of light brown sugar

- 1 teaspoon of vanilla extract

- 1/3 cup of fat-free milk

- Liquid stevia extract, to taste

Directions:

1. Preheat the oven to 350 °F and grease two 24-cup mini muffin pans with cooking spray.

2. Whisk together the flour, baking powder, baking soda, cinnamon, pumpkin pie spice, and salt in a large mixing bowl.

3. In a separate bowl, whisk together the eggs, pumpkin, applesauce, brown sugar, vanilla extract, and milk.

4. Stir the wet ingredients into the dry ones until well blended.

5. Adjust sweetness to taste with liquid stevia extract, if desired.

6. Spoon the batter into 36 cups and bake for 12 to 15 minutes until cooked through.

Nutrition:

- Calories: 35

- Total Fat: 13.6g

- Saturated Fat: 1.2g

- Total Carbs: 5.3g

- Net Carbs: 2.2g

- Protein: 5g

- Sugar: 1g

- Fiber: 3.1g

- Sodium: 53mg

Homemade Muffins

Preparation Time: 10 minutes

Cooking Time: 15 minutes

Servings: 3

Ingredients:

- 6 tbsp. of olive oil

- 100g of sugar

- 2 eggs

- 100g of flour

- 1 tsp. of Royal baking powder

- Lemon zest

Directions:

1. Beat the eggs with the sugar, with the help of a whisk. Add the oil little by little while stirring until you get a fluffy cream.

2. Then add the lemon zest.

3. Finally, add the sifted flour with the yeast to the previous mixture and mix in an envelope.

4. Fill 2/3 of the muffin baking tray with the dough.

5. Preheat the Air Fryer a few minutes to 180 °C, and when ready, place the muffins in the basket.

6. Set the timer for approximately 20 minutes at a temperature of 180 °C, until they are golden brown.

Nutrition:

- Calories: 240

- Fat: 12g

- Carbohydrates: 29g

- Protein: 4g

- Sugar: 100g

- Cholesterol: 67g

Chocolate and Nut Cake

Preparation Time: 10 minutes

Cooking Time: 30 minutes

Servings: 4

Ingredients:

- 60g of dark chocolate

- 2 butter spoons

- 1 egg

- 3 spoonful's of sugar

- 50g flour

- 1 envelope of Royal yeast

- Chopped walnuts

Direction:

1. Melt the dark chocolate with the butter over low heat. Once melted, put in a bowl.

2. Mix the egg, sugar, flour, yeast (the latter passed through the sieve to prevent lumps from forming), and finally, the chopped nuts.

3. Beat well by hand until you get a uniform dough.

4. Put the dough in a silicone mold or oven suitable for incorporation in the Air Fryer's basket.

5. Preheat the Air Fryer a few minutes at 180 ºC.

6. Set the timer for 20 minutes at 180 ºC, and when it has cooled down, unmold.

Nutrition:

- Calories: 108

- Fat: 12g

- Carbohydrates: 29g

- Protein: 4g

- Sugar: 100g

- Cholesterol: 3g

Chapter 6. Snacks Recipes

Sweet Potato Fries

Preparation Time: 5 minutes

Cooking Time: 13 minutes

Servings: 4

Ingredients:

- 2 medium sweet potatoes, peeled

- 1 tablespoon of arrowroot starch

- 2 tablespoons of cinnamon

- 1/4 cup of coconut sugar

- 2 teaspoons of melted butter, unsalted

- ½ tablespoon of olive oil

- Confectioner's swerve as needed

Directions:

1. Switch on the Air Fryer, insert fryer basket, grease it with olive oil, then shut with its lid, set the fryer to 370°F, and preheat for 5 minutes.

2. Meanwhile, cut peeled sweet potatoes into ½-inch thick slices, place them in a bowl, add oil and starch and toss until well coated.

3. Open the fryer, add sweet potatoes to it, close with its lid, and cook for 8 minutes until nicely golden, shaking halfway through the frying.

4. When the Air Fryer beeps, open its lid, transfer sweet potato fries in a bowl, add butter, sprinkle with sugar and cinnamon and toss until well mixed.

5. Sprinkle confectioners swerve on the fries and serve.

Nutrition:

- Calories: 130 Cal

- Carbs: 27 g

- Fat: 2.3 g

- Protein: 1.2 g

- Fiber: 3 g

Cheese Sticks

Preparation Time: 5-7 minutes

Cooking Time: 10 minutes

Serves: 2

Ingredients:

- 10 pieces of spring roll wrappers, separated, quartered

- ¼ pound of sharp cheddar cheese, reduced-fat, sliced into 2" x ½" matchsticks

- Oil for spraying

Directions:

1. Preheat the Air Fryer to 400°F.

2. Place cheese matchstick at the widest end of quartered spring roll wrapper. Moisten edges and tip of the wrapper with water. Fold spring roll wrapper over cheese, and tuck in both ends. Roll spring rolls tightly up to the tip. Place this into a freezer-safe container lined with saran wrap. Repeat the step for all cheese and spring roll wrappers.

3. Freeze for an hour before frying.

4. Spray a small amount of oil all over cheese matchsticks. Place a generous handful inside the Air Fryer basket. Fry for 3 to 5 minutes, or only until wrappers turn golden brown. Shake contents of the basket once midway through.

5. Remove from the basket. Set on plates. Repeat the step for the remaining breaded cheese sticks. Serve.

Nutrition:

- Calories: 229

- Carbohydrate: 16g

- Fat: 10g

- Protein: 15g

- Fiber: 1.8g

Zucchini Crisps

Preparation Time: 30 minutes

Cooking Time: 1 hour

Serves: 2

Ingredients:

- 2 zucchini, sliced into a 1/8-inch thick disk

- pinch of sea salt

- white pepper to taste

- olive oil for drizzling

Directions:

1. Preheat the Air Fryer to 330°F.

2. Put zucchini in a bowl with salt. Let it sit in a colander to drain for 30 minutes.

3. Layer zucchini in a baking dish. Drizzle in oil. Season with pepper. Place baking dish in the Air Fryer basket. Cook for 30 minutes.

4. Adjust seasoning. Serve.

Nutrition:

- Calories: 15.2

- Carbohydrate: 3.6g

- Fat: 0.1g

- Protein: 0.6g

- Fiber: 1.3g

Tortillas in Green Mango Salsa

Preparation Time: 30 minutes

Cooking Time: 10 minutes

Serves: 4

Ingredients:

Tortillas:

- 4 pieces of corn tortillas

- 1 tbsp. of olive oil

- 1/16 tsp. of sea salt

Green mango salsa:

- 1 green/unripe mango, minced

- 1 red/ripe Roma tomato, preferably minced

- 1 shallot, peeled, minced

- 1 fresh jalapeno pepper, minced

- ¼ red bell pepper, minced

- 4 tbsp. of fresh cilantro, minced

- ¼ cup of lime juice, freshly squeezed

- 1/16 tsp. of salt

Directions:

1. Preheat the Air Fryer to 400°F.

2. Mix lime juice and salt in a bowl. Stir until solids dissolve. Add in the remaining salsa ingredients. Chill in the fridge for at least 30 minutes. Stir again just before using.

3. Lightly brush oil on both sides of tortillas. Cut these into large triangles.

4. Place a generous handful of sliced tortillas in the Air Fryer basket. Fry these for 10 minutes or until bread blisters and turns golden brown. Shake contents of the basket once midway through.

5. Place cooked pieces on a plate. Repeat step for remaining tortillas. Season with salt.

6. Place equal portions of crispy tortillas on plates. Serve with green mango and tomato salsa on the side.

Nutrition:

- Calories: 128

- Carbohydrate: 8.6g

- Fat: 3.6g

- Protein: 2.7g

- Fiber: 5.7g

Skinny Pumpkin Chips

Preparation Time: 20 minutes

Cooking Time: 10 minutes

Servings: 2

Ingredients

- 1 pound pumpkin, cut into sticks
- 1 tablespoon coconut oil
- 1/2 teaspoon rosemary
- 1/2 teaspoon basil
- Salt and ground black pepper, to taste

Directions

1 Start by preheating the Air Fryer to 395 degrees F. Brush the pumpkin sticks with coconut oil; add the spices and toss to combine.

2 Cook for 13 minutes, shaking the basket halfway through the cooking time.

3 Serve with mayonnaise. Bon appétit!

Nutrition:

- 118 Calories; 7g
- Fat; 14.7g
- Carbs; 2.2g
- Protein; 6.2g Sugars

Palm Trees Holder

Preparation Time: 5 minutes

Cooking Time: 15 minutes

Servings: 2

Ingredients:

- 1 Sheet of puff pastry

- Sugar

Directions:

1. Stretch the puff pastry sheet.

2. Pour the sugar over and fold the puff pastry sheet in half.

3. Put a thin layer of sugar on top and fold the puff pastry in half again.

4. Roll the puff pastry sheet from both ends towards the center (creating the palm tree's shape).

5. Cut into sheets 5-8 mm thick.

6. Preheat the Air Fryer to 180 ºC and put the palm trees in the basket.

7. Set the timer about 10 minutes at 180 ºC.

Nutrition:

- Calories: 108

- Fat: 12g

- Carbohydrates: 29g

- Protein: 4g

- Sugar: 100g

- Cholesterol: 56g

Air Fried Ripe Plantains

Preparation Time: 10 minutes

Cooking Time: 10 minutes

Serves: 2

Ingredients:

- 2 pieces large ripe plantain, peeled, sliced into inch thick disks

- 1 Tbsp. of coconut butter, unsweetened

Directions:

1. Preheat the Air Fryer to 350 °F.

2. Brush a small amount of coconut butter on all sides of plantain disks.

3. Place one even layer into the Air Fryer basket, making sure none overlap or touch. Fry plantains for 10 minutes.

4. Remove from the basket. Place on plates. Repeat step for all plantains.

5. While plantains are still warm. Serve.

Nutrition:

- Calories: 209

- Carbohydrates: 29g

- Fat: 8g

- Protein: 2.9g

- Fiber: 3.5g

Garlic Bread with Cheese Dip

Preparation Time: 10 minutes

Cooking Time: 10 minutes

Serves: 8

Ingredients:

- Fried garlic bread

- 1 medium baguette, halved lengthwise, cut sides toasted

- 2 garlic cloves, whole

- 4 Tbsp. of extra virgin olive oil

- 2 Tbsp. of fresh parsley, minced

- Blue cheese dip

- 1 Tbsp. of fresh parsley, minced

- ¼ cup of fresh chives, minced

- ¼ tsp. of Tabasco sauce

- 1 Tbsp. of lemon juice, freshly squeezed

- ½ cup of Greek yogurt, low fat

- ¼ cup of blue cheese, reduced fat

- 1/16 tsp. of salt

- 1/16 tsp. of white pepper

Directions:

1. Preheat machine to 400°F.

2. Mix oil and parsley in a small bowl.

3. Vigorously rub garlic cloves on cut/toasted sides of the baguette. Dispose of garlic nubs.

4. Using a pastry brush, spread parsley-infused oil on the cut side of the bread.

5. Place the bread cut-side down on a chopping board. Slice into inch-thick half-moons.

6. Place bread slices in an Air Fryer basket. Fry for 3 to 5 minutes or until bread browns a little. Shake contents of the basket once midway through. Place cooked pieces on a serving platter. Repeat the step for the remaining bread.

7. To prepare blue cheese dip: mix all the ingredients in a bowl.

8. Place equal portions of fried bread on plates. Serve with blue cheese dip on the side.

Nutrition:

- Calories: 209

- Carbohydrates: 29g

- Fat: 8g

- Protein: 2.9g

- Fiber: 3.5g

Fried Mixed Veggies with Avocado Dip

Preparation Time: 10 minutes

Cooking Time: 10 minutes

Serves: 4

Ingredients

- Oil for spraying

Avocado-feta dip:

- 1 avocado, pitted, peeled, flesh scooped out

- 4 oz. of feta cheese, reduced fat

- 2 leeks, minced

- 1 lime, freshly squeezed

- ¼ cup of fresh parsley, chopped roughly

- 1/16 tsp. of black pepper

- 1/16 tsp. of salt

Vegetables:

- 1 zucchini, sliced into matchsticks

- 1 carrot, sliced into matchsticks

- 1 cup of panko breadcrumbs. Add more if needed

- 1 parsnip, sliced into matchsticks

- 1 large egg, whisked, add more if needed

- 1 cup of all-purpose flour, add more if needed

- 1/8 tsp. flaky sea salt

Directions:

1. Preheat the Air Fryer to 400°F.

2. Season carrots, parsnips, and zucchini with salt.

3. Dredge carrots with flour first, then dip them into the whisked egg, and finally into breadcrumbs. Place breaded pieces on a baking sheet lined with parchment paper. Repeat the step for all carrots. Then do the same for parsnips and zucchini.

4. Lightly spray vegetables with oil. Place a generous handful of carrots in the Air Fryer basket. Fry for 10 minutes or until breading turns golden brown, shaking contents of the basket once midway. Place cooked pieces on a plate. Repeat the step for the remaining carrots.

5. Do the previous step for parsnips and then zucchini.

6. For the dip, except for salt, place the remaining ingredients in a food processor. Pulse a couple of times, and then process to desired consistency scraping down sides of the machine often. Taste. Add salt only if needed. Place in an airtight container. Chill until needed.

7. Place equal portions of cooked vegetables on plates. Serve with a small amount of avocado-feta dip on the side.

Nutrition:

- Calories: 109

- Carbohydrates: 4.0g

- Fat: 2.6g

- Protein: 2.9g

- Fiber: 2.5g

Air Fried Plantains in Coconut Sauce

Preparation Time: 10 minutes

Cooking Time: 10 minutes

Servings: 8

Ingredients:

- 6 ripe plantains, peeled, quartered lengthwise

- 1 can of coconut cream

- 1 Tbsp. of Splenda

Directions:

1. Preheat the Air Fryer to 330°F.

2. Pour coconut cream in a thick-bottomed saucepan set over high heat; bring to boil. Reduce heat to lowest setting; simmer uncovered until the cream is reduced by half and darkens in color. Turn off heat.

3. Whisk in honey until smooth. Cool completely before using. Lightly grease a non-stick skillet with coconut oil.

4. Layer plantains in the Air Fryer basket and fry until golden on both sides; drain on paper towels. Place plantain into plates.

5. Drizzle in a small amount of coconut sauce. Serve.

Nutrition:

- Calories: 236

- Carbohydrates: 0g

- Fat: 1.5g

- Protein: 1g

- Fiber: 1.8g

Beef and Mango Skewers

Preparation Time: 10 minutes

Cooking Time: 4-7 minutes

Servings: 4

Ingredients:

- ¾ pound (340 g) of beef sirloin tip, cut into 1-inch cubes

- 2 tablespoons of balsamic vinegar

- 1 tablespoon of olive oil

- 1 tablespoon of honey

- ½ teaspoon of dried marjoram

- Pinch salt

- Freshly ground black pepper, to taste

- 1 mango

Directions:

1. Put the beef cubes in a medium bowl and add the balsamic vinegar, olive oil, honey, marjoram, salt, and pepper. Mix well, then rub the marinade into the beef with your hands. Set aside.

2. To prepare the mango, stand it on end and cut the skin off, using a sharp knife. Then carefully cut around the oval pit to remove the flesh. Cut the mango into 1-inch cubes.

3. Thread metal skewers alternating with three beef cubes and two mango cubes. Place the skewers in the Air Fryer basket.

4. Air fry at 390 ºF (199 ºC) for 4 to 7 minutes or until the beef is browned and at least 145 ºF (63 ºC).

Nutrition:

- Calories: 245

- Fat: 9g

- Protein: 26g

- Carbs: 15g

- Fiber: 1g

- Sugar: 14g

- Sodium: 96mg

Kale Chips with Lemon Yogurt Sauce

Preparation Time: 10 minutes

Cooking Time: 5 minutes

Servings: 4

Ingredients:

- 1 cup of plain Greek yogurt

- 3 tablespoons of freshly squeezed lemon juice

- 2 tablespoons of honey mustard

- ½ teaspoon of dried oregano

- 1 bunch of curly kale

- 2 tablespoons of olive oil

- ½ teaspoon of salt

- 1/8 teaspoon of pepper

Directions:

1. In a small bowl, mix the yogurt, lemon juice, honey mustard, and oregano, and set aside.

2. Remove the stems and ribs from the kale with a sharp knife. Cut the leaves into 2- to 3-inch pieces.

3. Toss the kale with olive oil, salt, and pepper. Rub the oil into the leaves with your hands.

4. Air fry the kale in batches at 390ºF (199ºC) until crisp, about 5 minutes, shaking the basket once during cooking time. Serve with the yogurt sauce.

Nutrition:

- Calories: 155

- Fat: 8g

- Protein: 8g

- Carbs: 13g

- Fiber: 1g

- Sugar: 3g

- Sodium: 378mg

Basil Pesto Bruschetta

Preparation Time: 10 minutes

Cooking Time: 4-8 minutes

Servings: 4

Ingredients:

- 8 slices of French bread, ½ inch thick

- 2 tablespoons of softened butter

- 1 cup of shredded Mozzarella cheese

- ½ cup of basil pesto

- 1 cup of chopped grape tomatoes

- 2 green onions, thinly sliced

Directions:

1. Spread the bread with the butter and place butter-side up in the Air Fryer basket. Bake at 350ºF (177ºC) for 3 to 5 minutes or until the bread is light golden brown.

2. Remove the bread from the basket and top each piece with some of the cheese. Return to the basket in batches and bake until the cheese melts, about 1 to 3 minutes.

3. Meanwhile, combine the pesto, tomatoes, and green onions in a small bowl.

4. When the cheese has melted, remove the bread from the Air Fryer and place on a serving plate. Top each slice with some of the pesto mixture and serve.

Nutrition:

- Calories: 463

- Fat: 25g

- Protein: 19g

- Carbs: 41g

- Fiber: 3g

- Sugar: 2g

- Sodium: 822mg

Cinnamon Pear Chips

Preparation Time: 15 minutes

Cooking Time: 9-13 minutes

Servings: 4

Ingredients:

- 2 firm Bosc pears, cut crosswise into 1/8 inch-thick slices

- 1 tablespoon of freshly squeezed lemon juice

- ½ teaspoon of ground cinnamon

- 1/8 teaspoon of ground cardamom or ground nutmeg

Directions:

1. Separate the smaller stem-end pear rounds from the larger rounds with seeds. Remove the core and seeds from the larger slices. Sprinkle all slices with lemon juice, cinnamon, and cardamom.

2. Put the smaller chips into the Air Fryer basket. Air fry at 380ºF (193ºC) for 3 to 5 minutes, until light golden brown, shaking the basket once during cooking. Remove from the Air Fryer.

3. Repeat with the larger slices, air frying for 6 to 8 minutes, until light golden brown, shaking the basket once during cooking.

4. Remove the chips from the Air Fryer. Cool and serve or store in an airtight container at room temperature up for to 2 days.

Nutrition:

- Calories: 31

- Fat: 0g

- Protein: 7g

- Carbs: 8g

- Fiber: 2g

- Sugar: 5g

- Sodium: 0mg

Phyllo Vegetable Triangles

Preparation Time: 15 minutes

Cooking Time: 6 to 11 minutes

Servings: 6

Ingredients:

- 3 tablespoons of minced onion

- 2 garlic cloves, minced

- 2 tablespoons of grated carrot

- 1 teaspoon of olive oil

- 3 tablespoons of frozen baby peas, thawed

- 2 tablespoons of nonfat cream cheese, at room temperature

- 6 sheets of frozen phyllo dough, thawed

- Olive oil spray, for coating the dough

Directions:

1. In a baking pan, combine the onion, garlic, carrot, and olive oil. Air fry at 390ºF (199ºC) for 2 to 4 minutes, or until the vegetables are crisp-tender. Transfer to a bowl.

2. Stir in the peas and cream cheese to the vegetable mixture. Let it cool while you prepare the dough.

3. Lay one sheet of phyllo on a work surface and lightly spray with olive oil spray. Top with another sheet of phyllo. Repeat with the remaining 4 phyllo sheets; you'll have 3 stacks with 2 layers each. Cut each stack lengthwise into 4 strips (12 strips total).

4. Place a scant 2 teaspoons of the filling near the bottom of each strip. Bring one corner up over the filling to make a triangle; continue folding the triangles over, as you would fold a flag. Seal the edge with a bit of water. Repeat with the remaining strips and filling.

5. Air fry the triangles, in 2 batches, for 4 to 7 minutes, or until golden brown. Serve.

Nutrition:

- Calories: 67

- Fat: 2g

- Protein: 2g

- Carbs: 11g

- Fiber: 1g

- Sugar: 1g

- Sodium: 121mg

Red Cabbage and Mushroom Pot Stickers

Preparation Time: 12 minutes

Cooking Time: 11-18 minutes

Servings: 12 pot stickers

Ingredients:

- 1 cup of shredded red cabbage

- ¼ cup of chopped button mushrooms

- ¼ cup of grated carrot

- 2 tablespoons of minced onion

- 2 garlic cloves, minced

- 2 teaspoons of grated fresh ginger

- 12 gyoza/pot sticker wrappers

- 2½ teaspoons of olive oil, divided

Directions:

1. In a baking pan, combine the red cabbage, mushrooms, carrot, onion, garlic, and ginger. Add 1 tablespoon of water. Place in the Air Fryer and bake at 370ºF (188ºC) for 3 to 6 minutes, until the vegetables are crisp-tender. Drain and set aside.

2. Working one at a time, place the pot sticker wrappers on a work surface. Top each wrapper with a scant 1 tablespoon of the filling. Fold half of the wrapper over the other half to form a half circle. Dab one edge with water and press both edges together.

3. To the baking pan, add 1¼ teaspoons of olive oil. Put half of the pot stickers, seam-side up, in the pan. Air fry for 5 minutes, or until the bottoms are light golden brown. Add 1 tablespoon of water and return the pan to the Air Fryer.

4. Air fry for 4 to 6 minutes more, or until hot. Repeat with the remaining pot stickers, remaining 1¼ teaspoons of oil, and another tablespoon of water. Serve immediately.

Nutrition:

- Calories: 88

- Fat: 3g

- Protein: 2g

- Carbs: 14g

- Fiber: 1g

- Sugar: 1g

- Sodium: 58mg

Garlic Roasted Mushrooms

Preparation Time: 3 minutes

Cooking Time: 22-27 minutes

Servings: 4

Ingredients:

- 16 garlic cloves, peeled

- 2 teaspoons of olive oil, divided

- 16 button mushrooms

- ½ teaspoon of dried marjoram

- 1/8 teaspoon of freshly ground black pepper

- 1 tablespoon of white wine cr low-sodium vegetable broth

Directions:

1. In a baking pan, mix the garlic with 1 teaspoon of olive oil. Roast in the Air Fryer at 350 ºF (177ºC) for 12 minutes.

2. Add the mushrooms, marjoram, and pepper. Stir to coat. Drizzle with the remaining 1 teaspoon of olive oil and the white wine.

3. Return to the Air Fryer and roast for 10 to 15 minutes more, or until the mushrooms and garlic cloves are tender. Serve.

Nutrition:

- Calories: 128

- Fat: 4g

- Protein: 13g

- Carbs: 17g

- Fiber: 4g

- Sugar: 8g

- Sodium: 20mg

Baked Spicy Chicken Meatballs

Preparation Time: 10 minutes

Cooking Time: 11-14 minutes

Servings: 24 meatballs

Ingredients:

- 1 medium red onion, minced

- 2 garlic cloves, minced

- 1 jalapeño pepper, minced

- 2 teaspoons of olive oil

- 3 tablespoons of ground almonds

- 1 egg

- 1 teaspoon of dried thyme

- 1 pound (454 g) of ground chicken breast

Directions:

1. In a baking pan, combine the red onion, garlic, jalapeño, and olive oil. Bake at 400ºF (204ºC) for 3 to 4 minutes, or until the vegetables are crisp-tender. Transfer to a medium bowl.

2. Mix in the almonds, egg, and thyme to the vegetable mixture. Add the chicken and mix until just combined.

3. Form the chicken mixture into about 24 (1-inch) balls. Bake the meatballs, in batches, for 8 to 10 minutes, until the chicken reaches an internal temperature of 165ºF (74ºC) on a meat thermometer.

Nutrition:

- Calories: 186

- Fat: 7g

- Protein: 29g

- Carbs: 5g

- Fiber: 1g

- Sugar: 3g

- Sodium: 55mg

Mini Onion Bites

Preparation Time: 10 minutes

Cooking Time: 16-20 minutes

Servings: 20 onion bites

Ingredients:

- 20 white boiler onions

- 1 cup of buttermilk

- 2 eggs

- 1 cup of flour

- 1 cup of whole-wheat bread crumbs

- 1 tablespoon of smoked paprika

- 1 teaspoon of salt

- 1 teaspoon of ground black pepper

- 1 teaspoon of granulated garlic

- ¾ teaspoon of chili powder

- Olive oil spray

Directions:

1. Place a parchment liner in the Air Fryer basket.

2. Slice off the root end of the onions, taking off as little as possible.

3. Peel off the papery skin and make cuts halfway through the tops of the onions. Don't cut too far down; you want the onion to hold together still.

4. In a large bowl, beat the buttermilk and eggs together.

5. In a medium bowl, mix the flour, bread crumbs, paprika, salt, pepper, garlic, and chili powder.

6. Add the prepared onions to the buttermilk mixture and allow to soak for at least 10 minutes.

7. Working in batches, remove the onions from the batter and dredge them with the bread crumb mixture.

8. Place the prepared onions in the Air Fryer basket in a single layer.

9. Spray lightly with the olive oil and air fry at 360ºF (182ºC) for 8 to 10 minutes, until golden and crispy. Repeat with any remaining onions and serve.

Nutrition:

- Calories: 166

- Fat: 2g

- Protein: 6g

- Carbs: 31g

- Fiber: 4g

- Sugar: 7g

- Sodium: 372mg

Crispy Parmesan Cauliflower

Preparation Time: 12 minutes

Cooking Time: 14 to 17 minutes

Servings: 20 cauliflower bites

Ingredients:

- 4 cups of cauliflower florets

- 1 cup of whole-wheat bread crumbs

- 1 teaspoon of coarse sea salt or kosher salt

- ¼ cup of grated Parmesan cheese

- ¼ cup of butter

- ¼ cup of mild hot sauce

- Olive oil spray

Directions:

1. Place a parchment liner in the Air Fryer basket.

2. Cut the cauliflower florets in half and set aside.

3. In a small bowl, mix the bread crumbs, salt, and Parmesan; set aside.

4. In a small microwave-safe bowl, combine the butter and hot sauce. Heat in the microwave until the butter is melted, about 15 seconds. Whisk.

5. Holding the stems of the cauliflower florets, dip them in the butter mixture to coat. Shake off any excess mixture.

6. Dredge the dipped florets with the bread crumb mixture, then put them in the Air Fryer basket. There's no need for a single layer; just toss them all in there.

7. Spray the cauliflower lightly with olive oil and air fry at 350ºF (177ºC) for 14 to 17 minutes, shaking the basket a few times throughout the cooking process. The florets are done when they are lightly browned and crispy. Serve warm.

Nutrition:

- Calories: 106

- Fat: 6g

- Protein: 3g

- Carbs: 10g

- Fiber: 1g

- Sugar: 1g

- Sodium: 416mg

Cream Cheese Stuffed Jalapeños

Preparation Time: 12 minutes

Cooking Time: 6-8 minutes

Servings: 10 poppers

Ingredients:

- 8 ounces (227 g) of cream cheese, at room temperature

- 1 cup of whole-wheat bread crumbs, divided

- 2 tablespoons of fresh parsley, minced

- 1 teaspoon of chili powder

- 10 jalapeño peppers, halved and seeded

Directions:

1. In a small bowl, combine the cream cheese, ½ cup of bread crumbs, the parsley, and the chili powder. Whisk to combine.

2. Stuff the cheese mixture into the jalapeños.

3. Sprinkle the tops of the stuffed jalapeños with the remaining ½ cup of bread crumbs.

4. Place in the Air Fryer basket and air fry at 360ºF (182ºC) for 6 to 8 minutes, until the peppers are softened, and the cheese is melted. Serve warm.

Nutrition:

- Calories: 244

- Fat: 16g

- Protein: 6g

- Carbs: 19g

- Fiber: 2g

- Sugar: 4g

- Sodium: 341mg

Parmesan French Fries

Preparation Time: 5 minutes

Cooking Time: 20-25 minutes

Servings: 16 fries

Ingredients:

- 2 russet potatoes, washed

- 1 tablespoon of olive oil

- 1 tablespoon of granulated garlic

- ¼ cup of grated Parmesan cheese

- ¼ teaspoon of salt

- ¼ teaspoon of ground black pepper

- 1 tablespoon of finely chopped fresh parsley (optional)

Directions:

1. Cut the potatoes into thin wedges and place in a large bowl.

2. Drizzle the olive oil over the potatoes, and toss to coat.

3. Sprinkle with the garlic, Parmesan cheese, salt, and pepper, and toss again.

4. Place in the Air Fryer basket and air fry at 400ºF (204ºC) for 20 to 25 minutes, until golden and crispy, stirring halfway through to ensure even cooking.

5. Top with the parsley (if using), and serve warm.

Nutrition:

- Calories: 209

- Fat: 5g

- Protein: 6g

- Carbs: 35g

- Fiber: 2g

- Sugar: 1g

- Sodium: 268mg

Cheesy Ham and Spinach Dip

Preparation Time: 8 minutes

Cooking Time: 7 minutes

Servings: 1 ½ cups

Ingredients:

- 8 ounces (227 g) of cream cheese

- 1 cup of shredded Cheddar cheese

- ½ cup of mayonnaise

- ¼ cup of Parmesan cheese

- 2 teaspoons of minced garlic

- 1 tablespoon of dried minced onion

- ½ cup of diced ham

- ½ cup of chopped fresh baby spinach

Directions:

1. In a large bowl, mix the cream cheese, Cheddar cheese, mayonnaise, Parmesan cheese, garlic, and dried minced onion. Use an electric mixer or a large wooden spoon to blend all the ingredients together.

2. Fold in the ham and spinach.

3. Transfer the mixture to a baking pan, and place in the Air Fryer basket.

4. Bake at 400ºF (204ºC) for 7 minutes, or until the cheese is melted, and serve.

Nutrition:

- Calories: 228

- Fat: 20g

- Protein: 8g

- Carbs: 4g

- Fiber: 0g

- Sugar: 1g

- Sodium: 398mg

Smoked Salmon Dip

Preparation Time: 10 minutes

Cooking Time: 7 minutes

Servings: 6

Ingredients:

- 1 (6-ounce / 170-g) can of boneless, skinless salmon

- 8 ounces (227 g) of cream cheese, softened

- 1 tablespoon of liquid smoke (optional)

- 1/3 cup of chopped pecans

- ½ cup of chopped green onions

- 1 teaspoon of kosher salt (or less if the salmon contains salt)

- 1 to 2 teaspoons of black pepper

- ¼ teaspoon of smoked paprika, for garnish

- Cucumber and celery slices, cocktail rye bread, or crackers

Directions:

1. In a baking pan, mix the salmon, softened cream cheese, liquid smoke (if using), pecans, ¼ cup of the green onions, and the salt and pepper. Stir until well combined.

2. Place the pan in the Air Fryer basket. Bake at 400ºF (204ºC) for 7 minutes, or until the cheese melts.

3. Sprinkle with the paprika and top with the remaining ¼ cup green onions. Serve with sliced vegetables, cocktail breads, or crackers.

Nutrition:

- Calories: 235

- Fat: 19g

- Protein: 13g

- Carbs: 3g

- Fiber: 0g

- Sugar: 1g

- Sodium: 650mg

Simple Corn Tortilla Chips

Preparation Time: 5 minutes

Cooking Time: 10 minutes

Servings: 4

Ingredients:

- 4 (6-inch) of corn tortillas

- 1 tablespoon of canola oil

- ¼ teaspoon of kosher salt

Directions:

1. Stack the corn tortillas, cut in half, then slice into thirds.

2. Spray the Air Fryer basket with nonstick cooking spray, then brush the tortillas with canola oil and place in the basket. Air fry at 360ºF (182ºC) for 5 minutes.

3. Pause the fryer to shake the basket, then air fry for 3 to 5 more minutes or until golden brown and crispy.

4. Remove the chips from the fryer and place on a plate lined with a paper towel. Sprinkle with the kosher salt on top before serving warm.

Nutrition:

- Calories: 72

- Fat: 4g

- Protein: 1g

- Carbs: 8g

- Fiber: 1g

- Sugar: 0g

- Sodium: 79mg

Chapter 7. Special Recipes

Asian Swordfish

Preparation Time: 10 Minutes

Cooking Time: 6 to 11 Minutes

Servings: 4

Ingredients:

- 4 (4-ounces) of swordfish steaks

- ½ teaspoon of toasted sesame oil (see Tip)

- 1 jalapeño pepper, finely minced

- 2 garlic cloves, grated

- 1 tablespoon of grated fresh ginger

- ½ teaspoon of Chinese five-spice powder

- 1/8 teaspoon of freshly ground black pepper

- 2 tablespoons of freshly squeezed lemon juice

Directions:

1. Place the swordfish steaks on a work surface and drizzle with the sesame oil.

2. In a small bowl, mix the jalapeño, garlic, ginger, five-spice powder, pepper, and lemon juice. Rub this mixture into the fish and let it stand for 10 minutes.

3. Roast the swordfish in the Air Fryer for 6 to 11 minutes, or until the swordfish reaches an internal temperature of at least 140°F on a meat thermometer. Serve immediately.

Nutrition:

- Calories: 187

- Fat: 6g (29% of calories from fat)

- Saturated Fat: 1g

- Protein: 29g

- Carbohydrates: 2g

- Sodium: 132mg

- Fiber: 0g

- Sugar: 1g

- 3% DV vitamin A

- 15% DV vitamin C

Full English Breakfast

Preparation Time: 30 minutes

Cooking Time: 30 minutes

Servings: 4

Ingredients:

- 8 Bacon Rashers

- 8 Sausages

- 10 oz. of Canned Baked Beans, drained

- 8 Medium Eggs

- 16 Cherry Tomatoes, halved

- 16 Button Mushrooms, halved

- Salt to taste

- Ground Black Pepper to taste

- 8 Toast Slices

Directions:

1. Put sausages and bacon in the Air Fryer, use the grill pan accessory if available, and cook them for 10 minutes at 360°F.

2. When done, transfer them to serving plates.

3. While sausages and bacon are cooking, take four 4 ounces ramekins and crack two eggs in each of them. Add salt and pepper to taste.

4. Pour beans in a 10 ounces ramekin, add salt and pepper.

5. Place both ramekins with eggs and beans in the Air Fryer and cook for 10 minutes at 400 °F.

6. Remove ramekins from the Air Fryer and place in it mushroom halves, and cook them for 6 minutes at 400°F.

7. Transfer eggs to the plates with bacon and sausages.

8. Stir beans and then spoon a quarter next to eggs on each plate.

9. Add the cherry tomatoes to the Air Fryer, sprinkle both mushrooms and tomatoes with salt and pepper to taste, and cook for another 4 minutes at 400°F.

10.   Divide tomatoes and mushrooms onto each plate.

11.   Enjoy!

Nutrition:

- Calories: 297

- Fat: 21.7g

- Carbs: 11.7g

- Protein: 15.3g

- Sugars: 2.6g

Country Breakie Chicken Tenders

Preparation Time: 10 minutes

Cooking Time: 15 minutes

Servings: 4

Ingredients:

- ¾ lb. of chicken tenders

For breading:

- 2 tablespoons of olive oil

- 1 teaspoon of black pepper

- ½ teaspoon of salt

- ½ cup of seasoned breadcrumbs

- ½ cup of all-purpose flour

- 2 eggs, beaten

Directions:

1. Preheat your Air Fryer to 330 ºF.

2. In three separate bowls, set aside breadcrumbs, eggs, and flour. Season the breadcrumbs with salt and pepper. Add olive oil to the breadcrumbs and mix well.

3. Place chicken tenders into flour, then dip into eggs, and finally dip into breadcrumbs. Press to ensure that the breadcrumbs are evenly coating the chicken. Shake off excess breading in the cooking basket. Cook the chicken tenders for 10-minutes in the Air Fryer. Serve warm.

Nutrition:

- Calories: 276

- Total Fat: 8.6g

- Carbs: 7g

- Protein: 13.2g

Greek Lamb Pita Pockets

Preparation Time: 15 minutes

Cooking Time: 5-7 minutes

Servings: 4

Ingredients:

Dressing:

- 1 cup of plain Greek yogurt

- 1 tablespoon of lemon juice

- 1 teaspoon of dried dill weed, crushed

- 1 teaspoon of ground oregano

- ½ teaspoon of salt

Meatballs:

- ½ pound (227 g) of ground lamb

- 1 tablespoon of diced onion

- 1 teaspoon of dried parsley

- 1 teaspoon of dried dill weed, crushed

- ¼ teaspoon of oregano

- ¼ teaspoon of coriander

- ¼ teaspoon of ground cumin

- ¼ teaspoon of salt

- 4 pita halves

Suggested Toppings:

- Red onion, slivered

- Seedless cucumber, thinly sliced

- Crumbled feta cheese

- Sliced black olives

- Chopped fresh peppers

Directions:

1. Stir all the dressing ingredients together and refrigerate while preparing lamb.

2. Mix all the meatball ingredients in a large bowl and stir to distribute seasonings.

3. Shape meat mixture into 12 small meatballs, rounded or slightly flattened if you prefer.

4. Air fry at 390ºF (199ºC) for 5 to 7 minutes, until well done. Remove and drain on paper towels.

5. To serve, pile meatballs and your choice of toppings in pita pockets and drizzle with dressing.

Nutrition:

- Calories: 270

- Fat: 14g

- Protein: 18g

- Carbs: 18g

- Fiber: 2g

- Sugar: 2g

- Sodium: 618mg

Asian Sesame Cod

Preparation Time: 5 minutes

Cooking Time: 7-9 minutes

Servings: 1

Ingredients:

- 1 tablespoon of reduced-sodium soy sauce

- 2 teaspoons of honey

- 1 teaspoon of sesame seeds

- 6 ounces (170 g) of cod fillet

Directions:

1. In a small bowl, mix the soy sauce and honey.

2. Spray the Air Fryer basket with nonstick cooking spray, then place the cod in the basket, brush with the soy mixture, and sprinkle sesame seeds on top. Roast at 360 ºF (182 ºC) for 7 to 9 minutes or until opaque.

3. Remove the fish from the fryer and let it cool on a wire rack for 5 minutes before serving.

Nutrition:

- Calories: 141

- Fat: 1g

- Protein: 26g

- Carbs: 7g

- Fiber: 1g

- Sugar: 6g

- Sodium: 466mg

Dijon Pork Tenderloin

Preparation Time: 10 minutes

Cooking Time: 12 to 14 minutes

Servings: 4

Ingredients:

- 1 pound (454 g) of pork tenderloin, cut into 1-inch slices

- Pinch salt

- Freshly ground black pepper, to taste

- 2 tablespoons of Dijon mustard

- 1 clove garlic, minced

- ½ teaspoon of dried basil

- 1 cup of soft bread crumbs

- 2 tablespoons of olive oil

Directions:

1. Slightly pound the pork slices until they are about ¾ inch thick. Sprinkle with salt and pepper on both sides.

2. Coat the pork with the Dijon mustard and sprinkle with the garlic and basil.

3. On a plate, mix the bread crumbs and olive oil and mix well. Coat the pork slices with the bread crumb mixture, patting so the crumbs adhere.

4. Place the pork in the Air Fryer basket, leaving a little space between each piece. Air fry at 390ºF (199ºC) for 12 to 14 minutes or until the pork reaches at least 145ºF (63ºC) on a meat thermometer and the coating is crisp and brown. Serve immediately.

Nutrition:

- Calories: 336

- Fat: 13g

- Protein: 34g

- Carbs: 20g

- Fiber: 2g

- Sugar: 2g

- Sodium: 390mg

Greek Chicken Kebabs

Preparation Time: 15 minutes

Cooking Time: 15 minutes

Servings: 4

Ingredients:

- 3 tablespoons of freshly squeezed lemon juice

- 2 teaspoons of olive oil

- 2 tablespoons of chopped fresh flat-leaf parsley

- ½ teaspoon of dried oregano

- ½ teaspoon of dried mint

- 1 pound (454 g) of low-sodium boneless, skinless chicken breasts, cut into 1-inch pieces

- 1 cup of cherry tomatoes

- 1 small yellow summer squash, cut into 1-inch cubes

Directions:

1. In a large bowl, whisk the lemon juice, olive oil, parsley, oregano, and mint.

2. Add the chicken and stir to coat. Let it stand for 10 minutes at room temperature.

3. Alternating the items, thread the chicken, tomatoes, and squash onto 8 bamboo or metal skewers that fit in an Air Fryer. Brush with marinade.

4. Air fry the kebabs at 380ºF (193ºC) for about 15 minutes, brushing once with any remaining marinade until the chicken reaches an internal temperature of 165ºF (74ºC) on a meat thermometer. Discard any remaining marinade. Serve immediately.

Nutrition:

- Calories: 164

- Fat: 4g

- Protein: 27g

- Carbs: 4g

- Fiber: 1g

- Sugar: 1g

- Sodium: 70mg

Scotch Eggs

Preparation Time: 10 minutes

Cooking Time: 15 minutes

Servings: 4

Ingredients:

- 1-pound of pork sausage, pastured

- 2 tablespoons of chopped parsley

- 1/8 teaspoon of salt

- 1/8 teaspoon of grated nutmeg

- 1 tablespoon of chopped chives

- 1/8 teaspoon of ground black pepper

- 2 teaspoons of ground mustard, and more as needed

- 4 eggs, hard-boiled, shell peeled

- 1 cup of shredded Parmesan cheese, low-fat

Directions:

1. Switch on the Air Fryer, insert fryer basket, grease it with olive oil, then shut with its lid, set the fryer at 400°F and preheat for 10 minutes.

2. Meanwhile, place sausage in a bowl, add salt, black pepper, parsley, chives, nutmeg, and mustard, then stir until well mixed and shape the mixture into four patties.

3. Peel each boiled egg, then place an egg on a patty and shape the meat around it until the egg has evenly covered.

4. Place cheese in a shallow dish, and then roll the egg in the cheese until covered completely with cheese; prepare remaining eggs the same way.

5. Then open the fryer, add eggs in it, close with its lid and cook for 15 minutes at the 400°F until nicely golden and crispy, turning the eggs and spraying with oil halfway through the frying.

6. When Air Fryer beeps, open its lid, transfer eggs onto a serving plate and serve with mustard.

Nutrition:

- Calories: 533 Cal

- Carbs: 2 g

- Fat: 43 g

- Protein: 33 g

- Fiber: 1 g

Chapter 8. 30 Day Meal Plan

Day	Breakfast	Lunch	Dinner
1	Pancakes	Parmesan Shrimp	Eggplant Surprise
2	Zucchini Bread	Tilapia	Carrots and Turnips
3	Blueberry Muffins	Tomato Basil Scallops	Shrimp and Asparagus
4	Baked Eggs	Shrimp Scampi	Instant Brussels sprouts with Parmesan
5	Bagels	Salmon Cakes	Braised Fennel
6	Cauliflower Hash Browns	Tex-Mex Salmon Stir-Fry	Brussels Sprouts & Potatoes Dish
7	Chicken Sandwich	Scallops with Green Vegetables	Beet and Orange Salad
8	Tofu Scramble	Cilantro Lime Shrimps	Endives Dish
9	Fried Egg	Juicy & Healthy Meatballs	Roasted Potatoes
10	Cheesecake Bites	Feta Lemon	Sugar Stuffed

		Meatballs	Bell Peppers
11	Coconut Pie	Cheesy Meatballs	Eggplant Surprise
12	Crust less Cheesecake	Honey Mustard Meatballs	Carrots and Turnips
13	Chocolate Cake	Greek Meatballs	Shrimp and Asparagus
14	Chocolate Brownies	Steak Burgers	Instant Brussels sprouts with Parmesan
15	Pancakes	Juicy Lamb Chops	Braised Fennel
16	Zucchini Bread	Lamb Roast	Brussels Sprouts & Potatoes Dish
17	Blueberry Muffins	Chicken in Tomato Juice	Beet and Orange Salad
18	Baked Eggs	Salmon on Bed of Fennel and Carrot	Endives Dish
19	Bagels	Roasted Vegetable Chicken Salad	Roasted Potatoes
20	Cauliflower Hash Browns	Warm Chicken and Spinach Salad	Sugar Stuffed Bell Peppers

21	Chicken Sandwich	Nutty Chicken Nuggets	Cabbage Wedges
22	Tofu Scramble	Spicy Chicken Meatballs	Buffalo Cauliflower Wings
23	Fried Egg	Chicken Wings with Curry	Sweet Potato Cauliflower Patties
24	Cheesecake Bites	Stuffed Chicken	Okra
25	Coconut Pie	Mesquite Pork Chops	Eggplant Surprise
26	Pancakes	Ranch Pork Chops	Carrots and Turnips
27	Zucchini Bread	Pork Chops with Peanut Sauce	Shrimp and Asparagus
28	Blueberry Muffins	Pork Spare Ribs	Instant Brussels sprouts with Parmesan
29	Baked Eggs	BBQ Pork Ribs	Braised Fennel
30	Bagels	Glazed Pork Shoulder	Brussels Sprouts & Potatoes Dish

Conclusion

Using an Air Fryer can be hard at first. If you follow our tips and tricks in this book, you will cook like a pro in no time! We have listed all sorts of recipes in this book so that you can make sure that you never run out of gas while trying to make your favorite foods again! Make sure to read through the whole book so that you can get everything right.

There's something about Air-fryers. When you think about it, they're kind of like a meal in a bit, without the hassle of actually cooking. All you have to do is grab a slice of bread or your favorite dish (or even a sandwich!), place it in the appliance, and wait for it to cook.

Air-fryers are convenient because they can be used at all hours. You can use them for cooking your favorite dish for dinner while you're getting ready or just for a quick snack in the middle of the day. You can even use them for cooking large meals such as breakfast foods or ethnic dishes overnight and saving yourself from having to clean up after dinner.

When you're using an Air-fryer, though, be careful about what foods you use. Some foods are difficult or impossible to fry when using an Air-fryer, so avoid using certain ingredients such as breaded chicken and pancakes with syrup or butter. There may be some other things you want to avoid, too, so be sure to check out our article on the diabetic Air-fryer cookbook.

The Diabetic Air-Fryer Cookbook provides a complete guide to using your air-fryer for the first time. In this section, you will learn everything you need to know about using your Air-fryer. It covers some basic information as well as advanced techniques.

This cookbook is designed to teach you some of the basics about how to use your Air-fryer, allowing you to enjoy all of its great features. We start with a shortlist of rules and tips that will help you make sure you are using your Air-fryer correctly. We also provide links in this section so that you can learn later if needed.

At Diabetic Air-Fryer Cookbook, we provide a full selection of accessories to help you use your Air-fryer more effectively. We provide an extensive selection of tools to repair your Air-fryer and make sure it is in a peak condition and last as long as possible.

After reading our cookbook, you'll find that we've covered all of the bases when it comes to using your Diabetic Air-Fryer Cookbook Air Fryer. You'll be able to cook healthy food every time with little effort and save money in the process! Make healthier choices without sacrifice from using this innovative and easy-to-use appliance!

This book will help you master the art of air frying and make your favorite meals completely pain-free and healthier than ever. One of the best ways to cook healthy food in a microwave is to use the air frying method. It involves cooking with steam, without oil or fats. This means that your kitchen will be free from a "fried" smell, and you can have a healthier diet.

This cookbook's contents will help you learn exactly how to do this by following step-by-step instructions that will be written for you without confusing words or often-used terms. We will teach you how to prepare and cook delicious and nutritious dishes quickly and easily when cooked using an Air Fryer. You can make breakfast, lunch, dinner, snacks, and desserts, so easily using this method. You will be able to prepare them in under 30 minutes without storing or freezing the ingredients because the foods are not fried at all.

It is just one of the key things that you can get from this book. Along with the "how-to" instructions, you will also receive helpful tips and tricks to help you when cooking with an Air Fryer.

CPSIA information can be obtained
at www.ICGtesting.com
Printed in the USA
BVHW011535100321
602204BV00010B/340

9 781801 920889